DIAGNOST

Pe

Dermatology

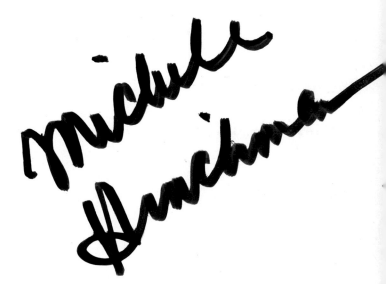

MW00736631

Prickly Heat:
- Avoid excess heat + humidity

- Light Clothing
- Cool Baths + AC
- Cetaphil Lotion or Aveeno Bar for cleaning Skin

DIAGNOSTIC PICTURE TESTS IN

Pediatric Dermatology

Julian Verbov MD, FRCP, FIBiol.
Consultant Paediatric Dermatologist
Royal Liverpool Children's Hospitals
Liverpool, England

M WOLFE

Titles published in the Diagnostic Picture Tests in . . . series include:

Picture Tests in Human Anatomy
DPT in Cardiology
DPT in Clinical Medicine, Vol 1–4
DPT in Clinical Neurology
DPT in Dermatology
DPT in Ear, Nose and Throat
DPT in Embryology
DPT in Endocrinology
DPT in Gastroenterology
DPT in General Dentistry
DPT in General Medicine
DPT in General Surgery
DPT in Geriatric Medicine
DPT in Infectious Diseases
Differential Diagnosis in AIDS

400 Self Assessment Picture Tests in
  Clinical Medicine
DPT in Injury in Sport
DPT in Obstetrics/Gynaecology
DPT in Ophthalmology
DPT in Oral Medicine
DPT in Orthopaedics
DPT in Paediatrics, 2nd edn
DPT in Paediatric Dentistry
DPT in Respiratory Disease
DPT in Rheumatology
DPT in Urology
400 More Self Assessment Picture
  Tests in Clinical Medicine

Copyright © 1994 Mosby–Year Book Europe Limited
Published in 1994 by Wolfe Publishing, an imprint of Mosby–Year Book Europe
Limited
Printed in Spain by Grafos, S.A. ARTE SOBRE PAPEL
ISBN 0 7234 1961 2

For full details of all Mosby–Year Book Europe Limited titles please write to
Mosby–Year Book Europe Limited, Lynton House, 7–12 Tavistock Square, London
WC1H 9LB, England.

A CIP catalogue record for this book is available from the British Library.

Library of Congress Cataloging-in-Publication Data has been applied for.

Acknowledgements

I should like to thank Mr David Adkins of the Royal Liverpool University Hospital Department of Medical Illustration and Mr Charles Fitz-Simon of the Royal Liverpool Children's Hospital, Alder Hey, Department of Medical Photography, for providing and allowing reproduction of many of the photographs in this book. I thank colleagues who have permitted me to use photographs of some of their patients. I should like to thank my dear wife for typing the manuscript.

Preface

This book is devoted to all those who deal with childhood disorders. It is for browsing through rather than reading at a sitting. Commonly referred conditions are emphasised and therefore atopic dermatitis, scabies, psoriasis, and viral infections feature prominently. However, uncommon and rare conditions, including some with systemic associations also find a place because it is important to recognise these. Answers are brief, but informative. Readers are encouraged to seek more detailed information in standard texts and current journals. Paediatricians, dermatologists in training, medical students, those studying for higher examinations and nursing personnel should all find much of interest.

Julian Verbov

Dedication

For my twin granddaughters

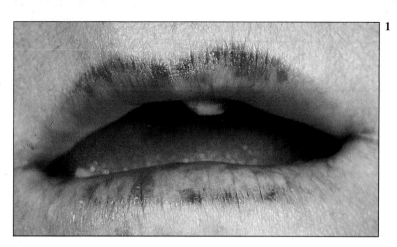

1 This child presented with abdominal pain and melaena.
(a) What is the diagnosis?
(b) Describe the features.
(c) How can you explain the presentation?

2 This baby was referred with an eruption in the napkin area.
(a) What is the cause?
(b) Describe the lesions.
(c) How would you treat this?

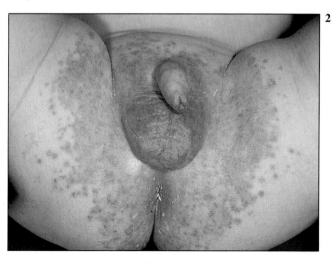

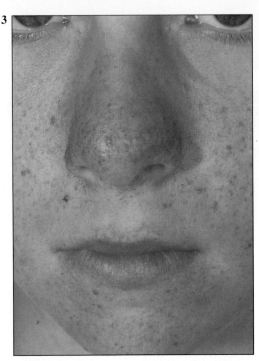

3, 4 This 12-year-old boy had a history of epilepsy.
(a) Can you make a diagnosis?
(b) Mention some other skin signs.
(c) What is the mode of inheritance?

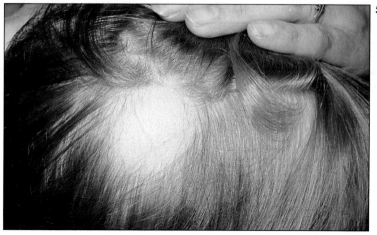

5 This is a common type of hair fall.
(a) What is it called?
(b) What is the cause?
(c) What is the prognosis?

6 This boy had a sore mouth followed by skin lesions.
(a) What is the condition?
(b) How are such lesions shown commonly described?
(c) Do you know any causes?
(d) What types are there?

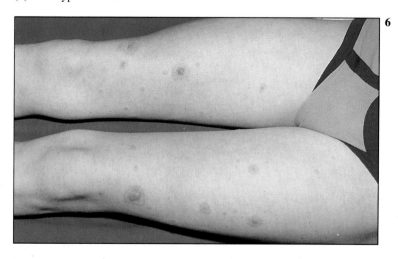

7

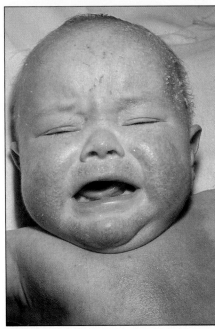

7 A 5-month-old infant with itchy skin since 3 months old.
(a) What is the diagnosis?
(b) What treatment would you advise?
(c) Comment on the prognosis.

8

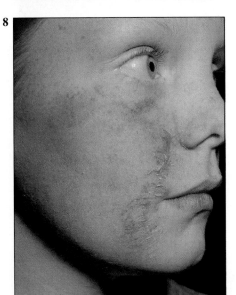

8 This girl presented with a tender swelling of the right cheek.
(a) What is the condition?
(b) How is it acquired?
(c) How would you treat it?

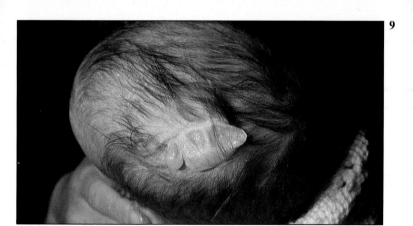

9 A 2-month-old infant presented with this asymptomatic unilateral left parietal lesion.
(a) What is the diagnosis?
(b) What is the differential diagnosis?
(c) How would you treat it?

10 This large lesion appeared within the first month of life.
(a) What is it called?
(b) What will happen to it?
(c) How would you manage it?

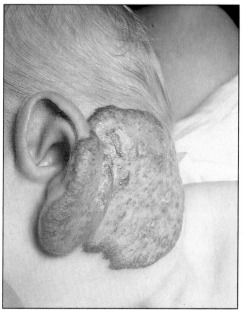

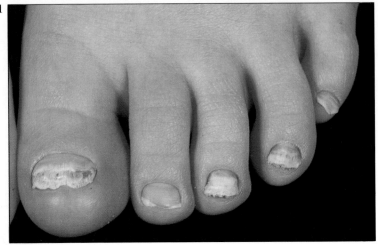

11 This 3-year-old boy presented with abnormal toenails.
(a) What is the diagnosis?
(b) How do you confirm the diagnosis?
(c) How would you treat him?

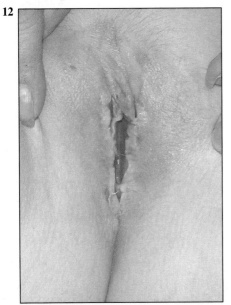

12 This prepubertal girl showed white perivulval patches initially.
(a) What is the diagnosis?
(b) What can you see?
(c) How do you treat it?
(d) What is the prognosis?

13 The boy shown had flesh-coloured lesions over his body and was itching.
(a) What is the diagnosis?
(b) Name some causes of the acute form.
(c) What is the treatment?

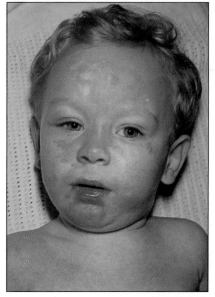

14 This eruption affected hands and feet and some contacts were also affected.
(a) What is the diagnosis?
(b) What can you see?
(c) What is the cause?
(d) What is the natural history?

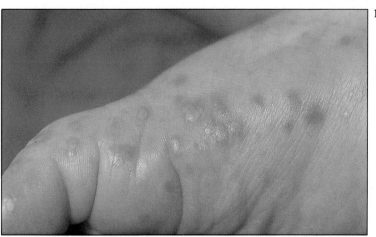

15 This child presented with discrete slaty-grey, asymptomatic patches over trunk and arms.
(a) What is this condition?
(b) What is the cause?

16 This 3-year-old presented with a sore mouth.
(a) What is the diagnosis?
(b) What can you see?
(c) How would you manage it?

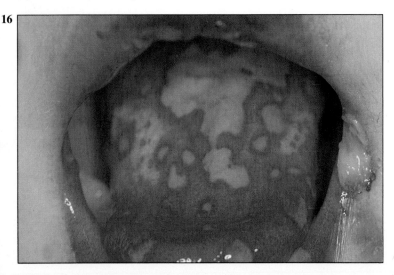

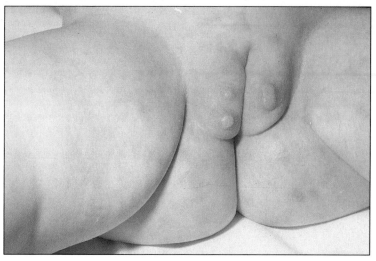

17 This is a 10-month-old infant with napkin area lesions.
(a) What is the diagnosis?
(b) Describe what you see.
(c) What is the cause of the lesions?

18 This is a Nigerian child.
(a) What do you call these patches?
(b) What do they indicate?
(c) What is the natural history of such lesions?

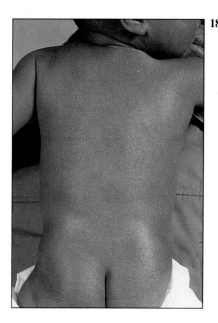

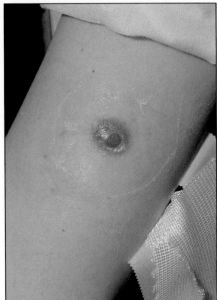

19, 20 The clinical pictures illustrate reactions to a vaccine injection.
(a) What is the vaccine?
(b) How would you describe the first lesion and how would you treat it?
(c) How would you describe the second and rarer reaction in which patches that ulcerated appeared around the injection site 6 months after vaccination, and how would you treat it?

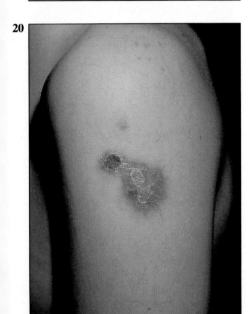

21 This is a 7-month-old boy.
(a) Describe the lesion.
(b) What are the likely causes?
(c) How would you treat him?

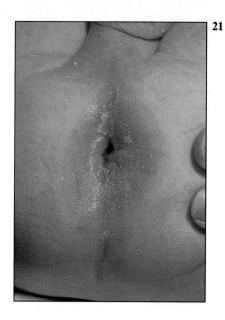

22 This unwell neonate presented with enlarging lesions.
(a) What is the diagnosis?
(b) What is the prognosis of this rare condition?

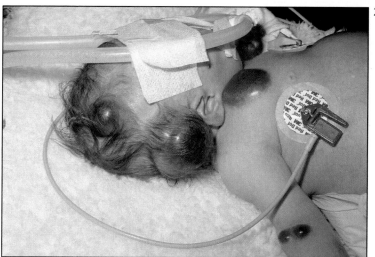

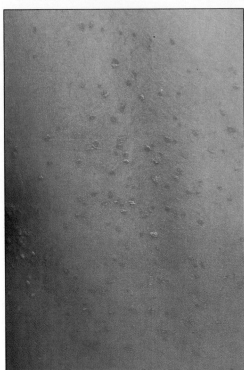

23 This is common in children.
(a) What is it?
(b) What is the natural history of the attack?
(c) How would you treat it?

24 The mother had the same condition as her 20-month-old daughter shows.
(a) What is it?
(b) What is the mode of inheritance?
(c) What are common signs?

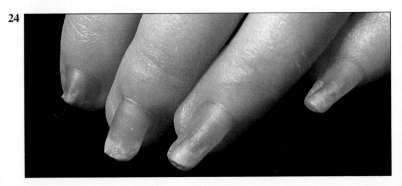

25 This is a pigmentation disorder
(a) What is it?
(b) What is the defect?
(c) Describe its management.

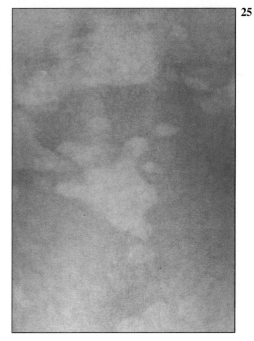

26 This non-palpable rash followed varicella.
(a) What is the diagnosis?
(b) What is the prognosis?

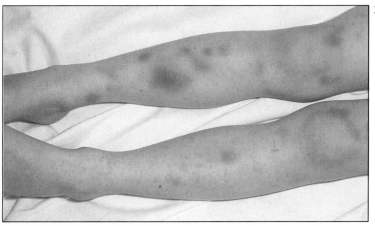

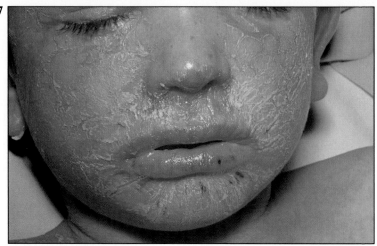

27, 28 This 4-year-old developed fever followed by a widespread scald-like eruption. His appearance both on admission and 4 days later with treatment are shown.
(a) What is this called?
(b) What is it due to?
(c) What is the treatment?

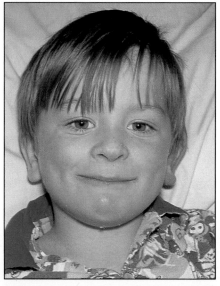

29 This 6-year-old child rapidly developed tight skin over the face and elsewhere.
(a) What is this uncommon condition?
(b) What is the cause?
(c) What are the clinical features?
(d) What is the prognosis?

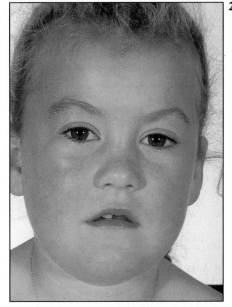

30 An eruption in a 7-year-old boy.
(a) What is the diagnosis?
(b) What is the incubation period?
(c) For how long does the child remain infectious?

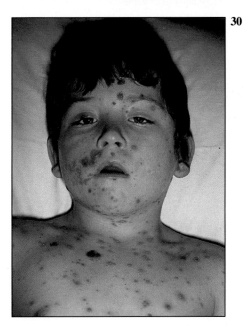

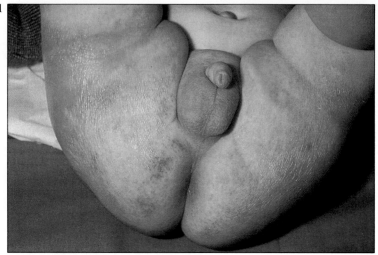

31 A napkin area eruption.
(a) What is the diagnosis?
(b) What does the convex area of involvement indicate?
(c) What is the treatment?

32 This 3-year-old boy has a widespread irritant eruption.
(a) What does the picture show?
(b) Would other family contacts be affected?
(c) What is the treatment?

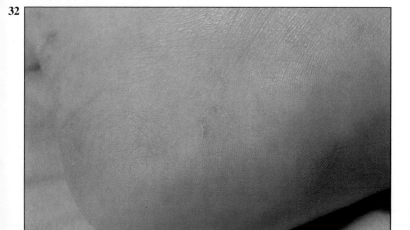

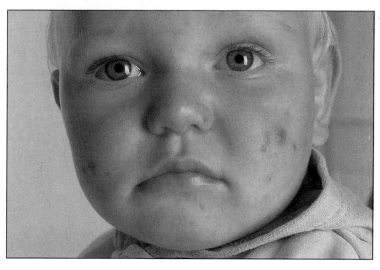

33 A 10-month-old boy.
(a) What has he got?
(b) Would you expect to find evidence of sexual precocity?
(c) What is the management?

34 Look at this boy's nails.
(a) What do they show?
(b) What is their significance?

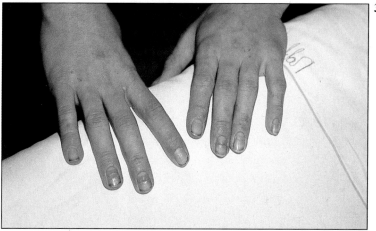

35

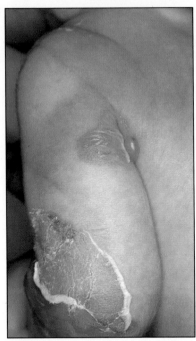

35, 36, 37 Three examples of a group of rare genetically determined non-inflammatory blistering disorders.
(a) What is the group called?
(b) How many types are there?
(c) At what level in the skin do the blisters occur?
(d) What is the most important part of management?

36

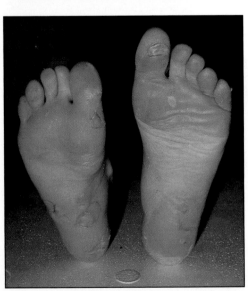

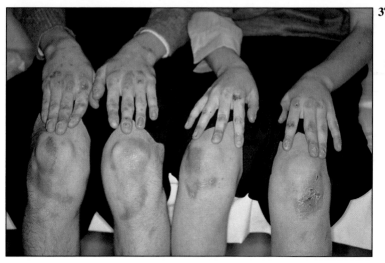

38 A 14-year-old girl.
(a) What is the lesion?
(b) Where do they develop?

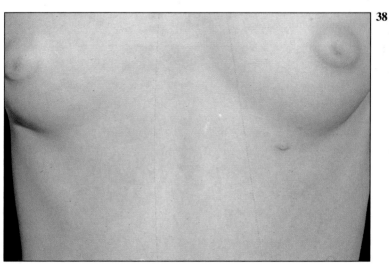

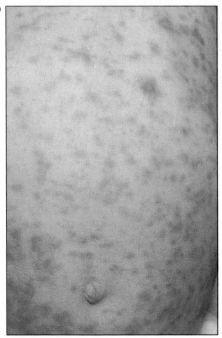

39 A widespread eruption in a 14-month-old boy.
(a) What is the diagnosis?
(b) Describe what you can see.
(c) What is the treatment?
(d) What is the prognosis?

40 Note the big toenails.
(a) What is the abnormality?
(b) What is its management?

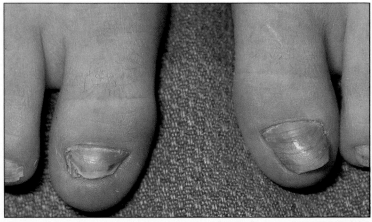

41 A congenital back lesion.
(a) What is it called?
(b) What do you do about it?

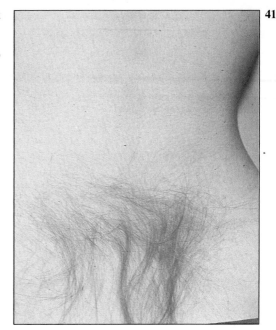

42 A common condition.
(a) What is the diagnosis?
(b) Why does it occur?

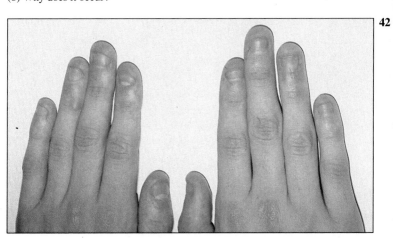

43

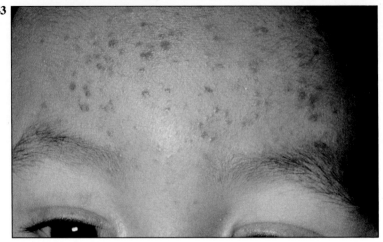

44

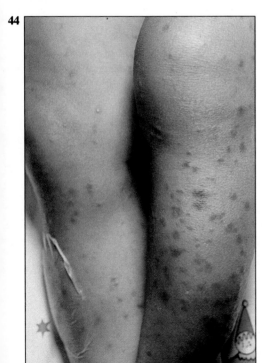

43, 44 A 6-month-old boy with an eruption over face, limbs, and buttocks, but sparing the trunk.
(a) What is the diagnosis?
(b) Describe the lesions.
(c) What are the causes?
(d) What is the prognosis?

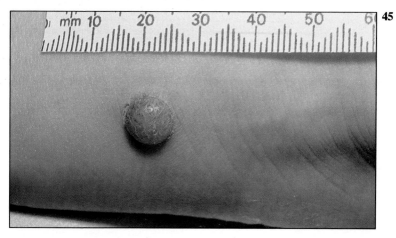

45 This is a foot nodule in a young girl.
(a) What is the diagnosis?
(b) Do they always look like this?
(c) How would you confirm the diagnosis?

46 This infant had an eruption
in both axillae.
(a) What is the diagnosis?
(b) How would you treat it?

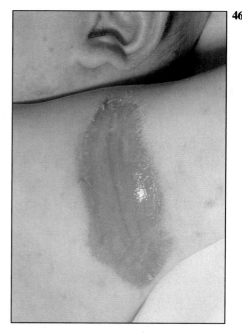

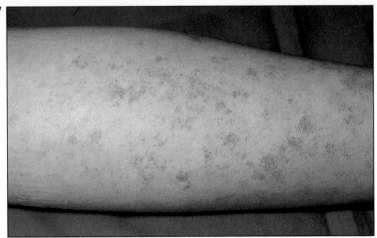

47 This child's uncommon eruption was unilateral and asymptomatic and occurred over both upper and lower limbs.
(a) What is the diagnosis?
(b) What is the prognosis?

48 A 15-year-old girl who had scalp hair loss associated with excessive thirst and polyuria.
(a) What was the cause of the hair loss?
(b) Did the hair regrow?

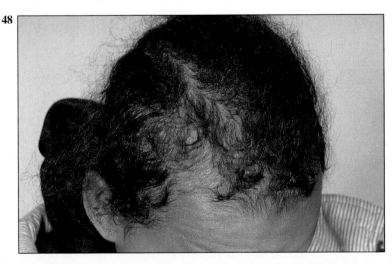

49 This infant developed this eruption, which also involved inner buttocks and scalp, soon after his mother stopped breast feeding.
(a) What is the diagnosis?
(b) What is the cause?
(c) What is the treatment?
(d) How else may the deficiency and skin signs arise?

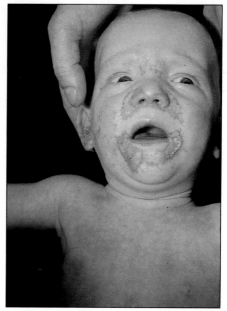

50 A 4-year-old boy with peri-anal lesions.
(a) What are they?
(b) How did he get them?
(c) What is the management?

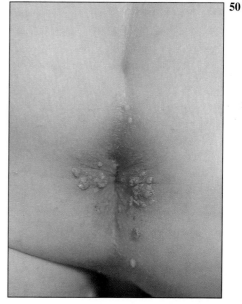

51

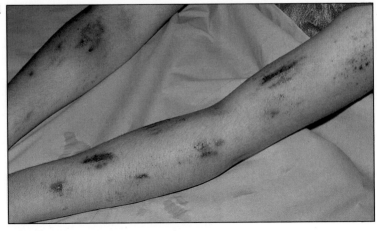

51 This girl complained of the sudden appearance of these lesions.
(a) What is the diagnosis?
(b) Why?
(c) Who tend to be affected by this condition?

52

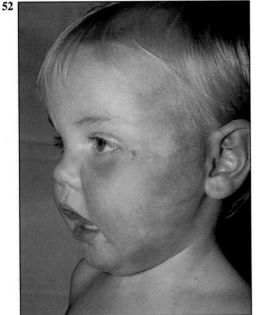

52 A parent brought this boy to the Accident and Emergency Department.
(a) What is the probable diagnosis?
(b) What would be your next step?

53 This 3-year-old girl's hair had always looked normal.
(a) What is the diagnosis?
(b) Describe the signs.
(c) What is the prognosis?

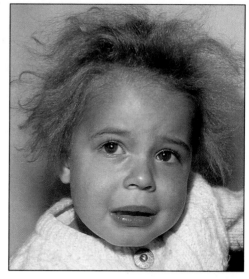

54 This is a common sign.
(a) What is shown?
(b) What does this sign indicate?

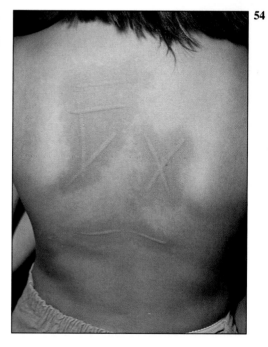

55

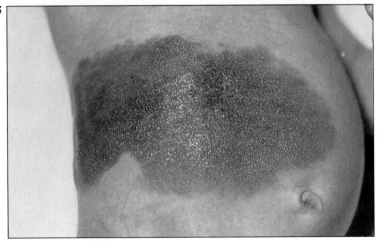

55 A 17-day-old neonate.
(a) What is the diagnosis?
(b) What is the management?

56

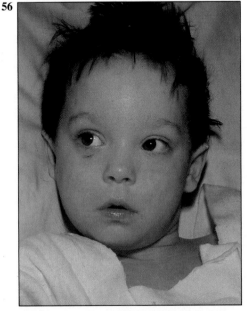

56 This 4-year-old boy presented with atopic-type eczema. He also had thrombocytopenia and a history of recurrent infections.
(a) What is the diagnosis?
(b) What is the mode of inheritance?
(c) What is the prognosis?

57 A common condition.
(a) What has this 1-year-old boy got?
(b) What is a common complication?

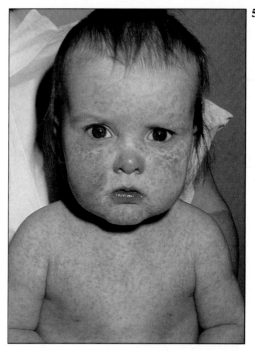

58 This shows the effect of big toe trauma.
(a) What is the diagnosis?
(b) How is it treated?

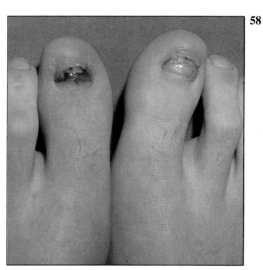

59

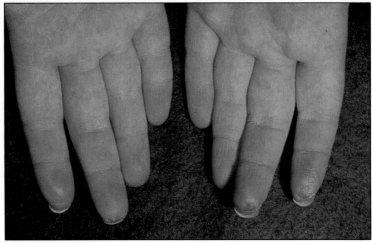

59 This young girl gave a history of cold hands.
(a) What diagnosis would you make?
(b) What are the changes described by the patient?
(c) What is the cause?

60 A 16-week-old infant with papules and vesicles over soles and palms.
(a) What is the diagnosis?
(b) What is the incubation period after infection?
(c) How would you confirm the diagnosis?

60

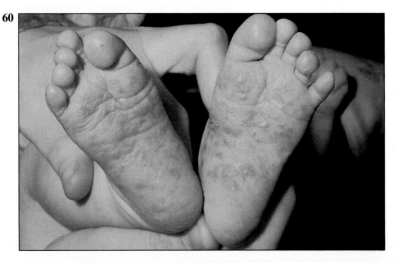

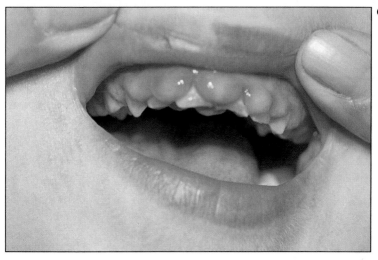

61 This 6-year-old developed this visible change when on a drug.
(a) What is the diagnosis?
(b) Can you name two drug causes?

62 This neonate has a blistering eruption.
(a) Can you make a diagnosis?
(b) Describe the clinical features.
(c) Are there any complications associated with this disorder?

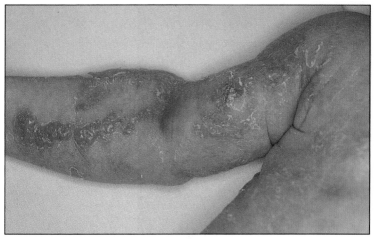

63

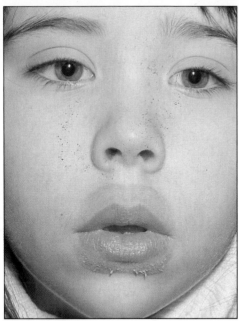

63 This common condition is often not recognised by parents and/or affected individuals.
(a) What is this child doing?
(b) Such children often have a certain diathesis. What is it?

64

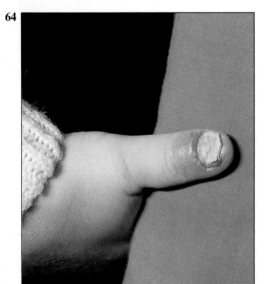

64 A relatively common problem.
(a) What is the diagnosis?
(b) In whom does it occur?

65 This 10-year-old girl has a scalp problem.
(a) What is the diagnosis?
(b) What are the causes?
(c) What is the treatment?

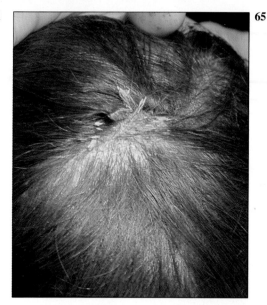

66 An uncommon, but striking, eruption.
(a) What is this well-defined lesion?
(b) What is the usual history?

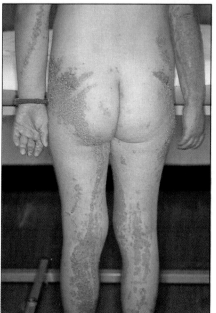

67

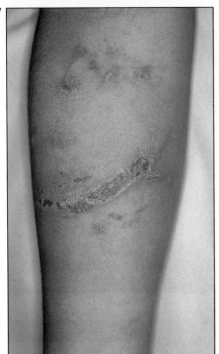

67 A linear painful blistering lesion was sustained at the site shown nine days earlier while swimming in the South of France.
(a) What is the likely diagnosis?
(b) What is the emergency treatment?

68 This 15-year-old girl also had joint hypermobility.
(a) What is the diagnosis?
(b) How many types are there?
(c) What is the common mode of inheritance?

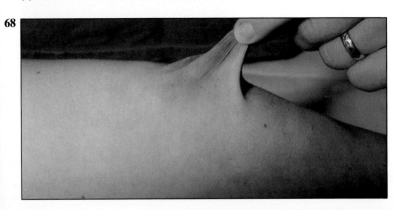

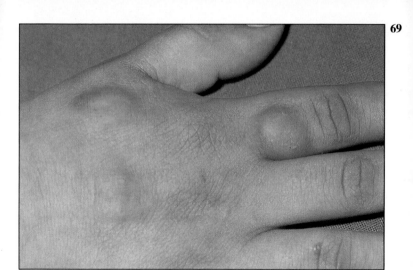

69 A well 10-year-old boy presented with these.
(a) What are they?
(b) How did they appear?

70 A bald patch had been pre-sent since birth.
(a) What is this called?
(b) Describe the complications.
(c) What is the management?

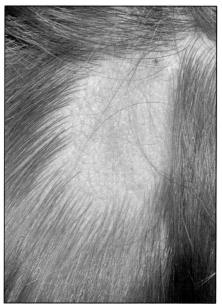

71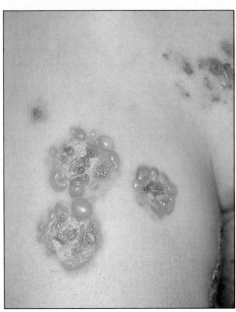

71 This striking characteristic eruption appeared in a 5-year-old.
(a) What is the diagnosis?
(b) How does it present?
(c) What is the treatment?
(d) What is its prognosis?

72 This 13-year-old girl gave a history of Raynaud's syndrome, weight loss, and weakness, and was noted to have a rather beaked nose.
(a) What is the diagnosis?
(b) How would you manage the patient?

72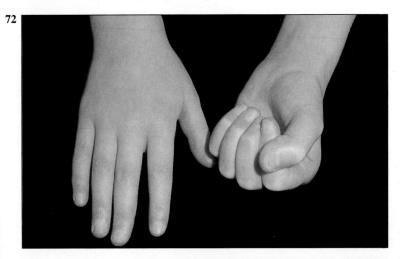

73 Overcrowding and poor hygiene may be relevant in this condition.
(a) What is the diagnosis?
(b) What causes it?
(c) How would you treat it?

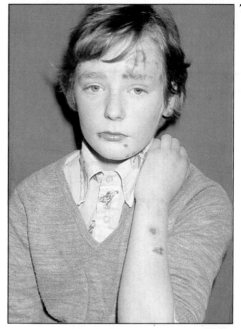

74 This is a rare dominant condition and this patient's sister was also affected. Note the symmetry of lower limb lesions.
(a) What is the diagnosis?
(b) What are the signs?

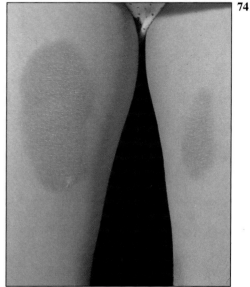

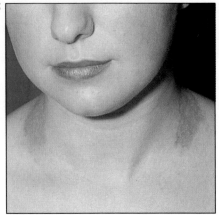

75 Surprisingly this girl denied wearing fashion jewellery.
(a) What is the likely diagnosis?
(b) How was this confirmed?

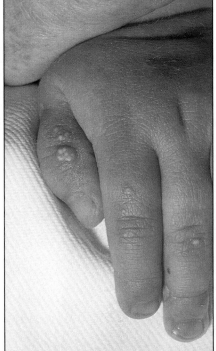

76 This fit child had hard papules as shown.
(a) Can you make a diagnosis?
(b) What are the causes of such deposition?

77 A 3-week-old child with a common condition.
(a) What is the diagnosis?
(b) How is it managed.

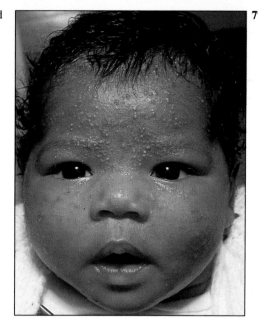

78 Notice the distribution of the eruption.
(a) What is the diagnosis?
(b) Where does it usually begin?
(c) What is its aetiology?

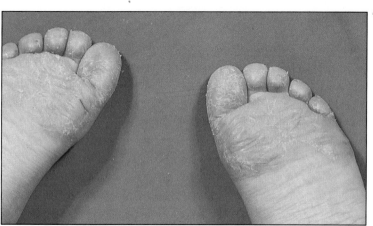

79

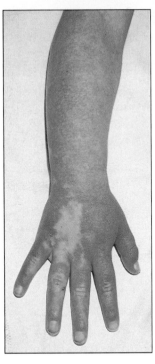

79 This congenital developmental defect is most common on the face.
(a) What is it called?
(b) Is there any treatment?
(c) What is the Sturge-Weber syndrome?

80

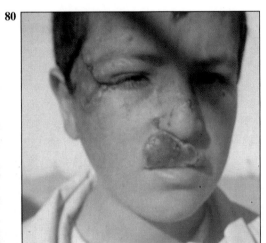

80 A 10-year-old Iranian boy.
(a) What is the probable diagnosis?
(b) What do you know about the condition?
(c) What is the cause?
(d) How can you prevent the complications?

48

81 This child has atopic dermatitis.
(a) What is this complication?
(b) What treatment do you advise?

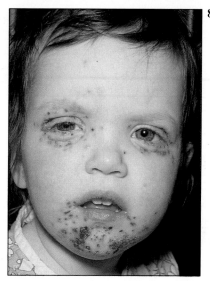

82 A rather florid chest lesion in a 6-year-old boy.
(a) Can you make a diagnosis?
(b) Describe the condition.
(c) What is the treatment?

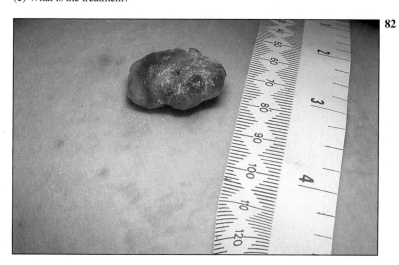

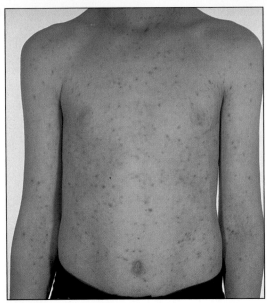

83, 84 This boy had a widespread rash.
(a) What is the diagnosis?
(b) What are the clinical features?
(c) How long does it last?

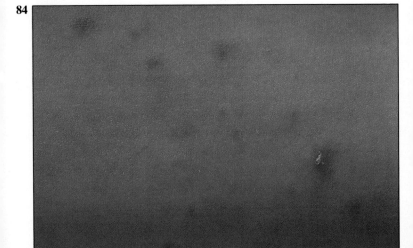

85 This common condition is easy to feel but not so easy to photograph.
(a) What is the diagnosis?
(b) What area does it affect?

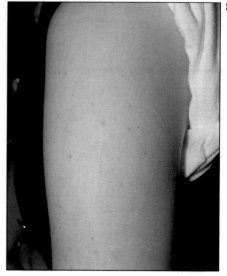

86 The photograph shows the feet of a mother and daughter with this inherited condition.
(a) What is the diagnosis?
(b) What is the mode of inheritance?
(c) Is it always a benign sign?

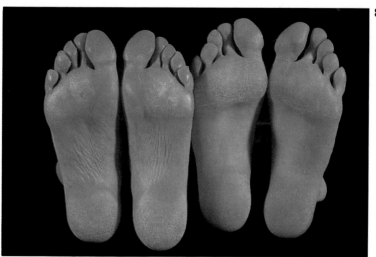

87 A cosmetically unsightly
lesion.
(a) What is it?
(b) What is its natural history?
(c) What is the management?

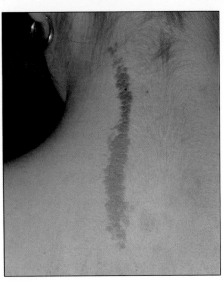

88 This is a 9-day-old girl.
(a) What has she got?
(b) What is the mode of inheritance?
(c) What are the most common types?
(d) How is it managed?

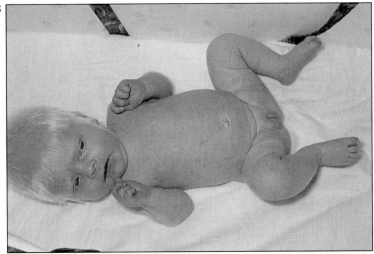

89, 90 This fit child presented with lesions on limbs and face.
(a) What is the diagnosis?
(b) What is the usual age of onset?
(c) What are the clinical features?
(d) What is the prognosis?

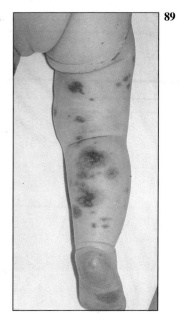

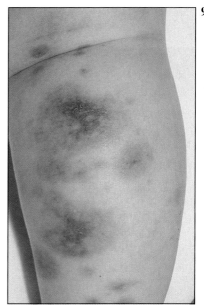

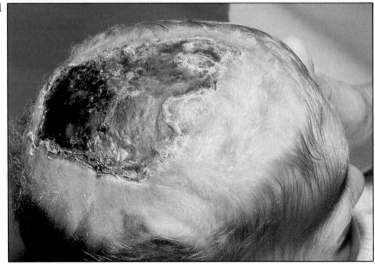

91, 92 This child was born with a scalp defect. The pictures were taken when 2 weeks old and 3 years old.
(a) What is the condition called?
(b) What does it affect?
(c) What are the complications?
(d) What is the routine management?

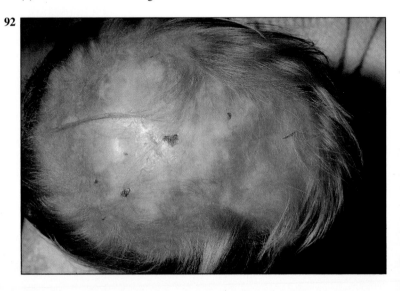

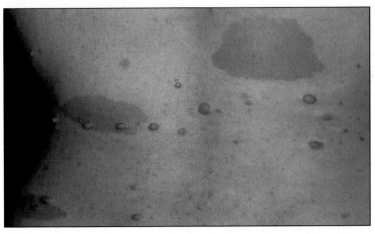

93 This patient is post-pubertal.
(a) What is the diagnosis?
(b) What are some of the manifestations?

94 This baby's mother had systemic lupus erythematosus.
(a) What is the condition?
(b) What are the usual signs?
(c) What are the serological markers?

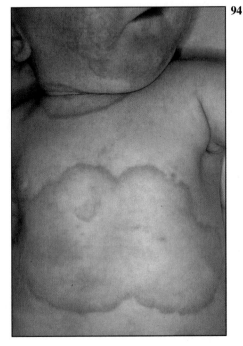

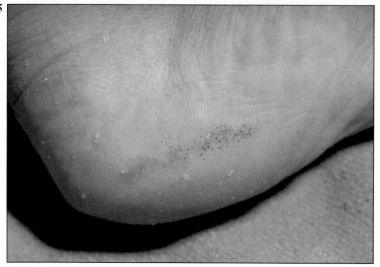

95 This heel shows a localised area of black spots.
(a) What is the condition?
(b) What is the cause?

96 These lesions are very common in children.
(a) What are they?
(b) What virus causes them?
(c) What is their natural history?

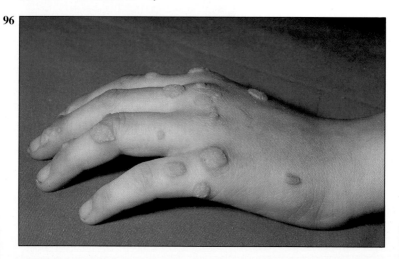

97 This condition usually begins in the first 3 months of life.
(a) What is it?
(b) What is lacking in this condition?
(c) How is it treated?

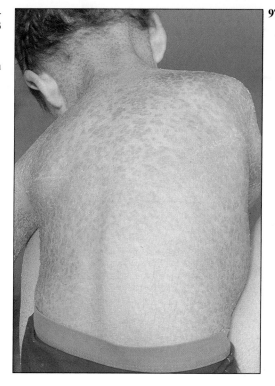

98 Most of this boy's nails were affected.
(a) What is this condition?
(b) Do you know any causes?
(c) What is the prognosis?

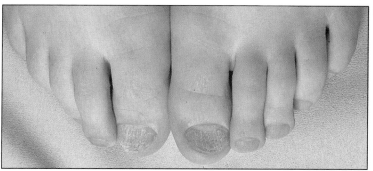

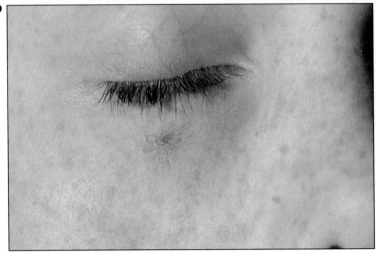

99 This lesion is unsightly rather than worrying.
(a) What is the diagnosis?
(b) Is it common?
(c) Can it be treated?

100 This 1-year-old infant developed blisters over the left side of the face.
(a) What is your diagnosis?
(b) How is the condition treated?

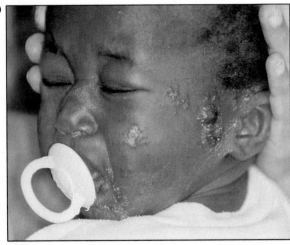

101, 102 Here are two infants with the same common condition.
(a) What is the diagnosis?
(b) What are the usual features?
(c) Can scalp involvement occur alone?

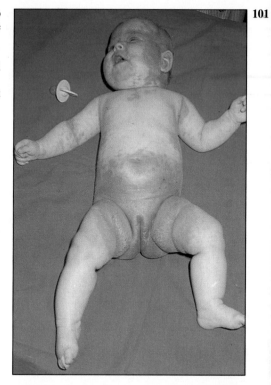

101

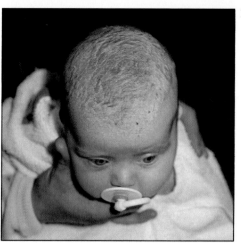

102

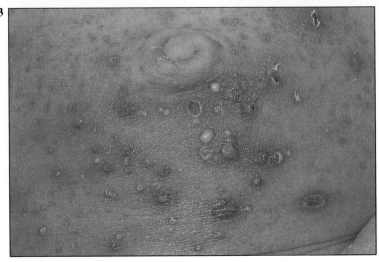

103 An important pustular eruption in a neonate.
(a) What is the diagnosis?
(b) What is the treatment?

104 This 4-year-old was left in the sun for a few hours with unprotected skin.
(a) What is the diagnosis?
(b) How is it treated?

105 A common condition.
(a) What is it?
(b) What lesions are usual?
(c) How is it managed?

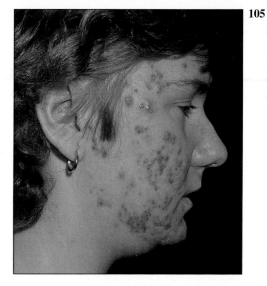

106 This child had hair loss
and strands could be pulled
out painlessly and easily.
(a) What is the diagnosis?
(b) What is the prognosis?

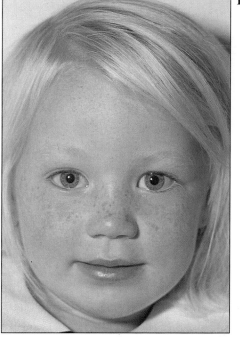

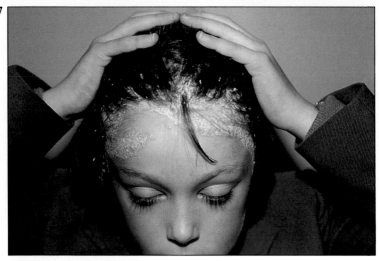

107 This boy had a widespread eruption as well.
(a) What is the diagnosis?
(b) How is the eruption on the scalp managed?

108 This condition in which affected areas feel like wooden blocks started in this well child when 18 days old.
(a) Can you make a diagnosis?
(b) What is the management?

109 Painful skin lesions, which were discrete at first.
(a) What is the diagnosis?
(b) What is the aetiology?

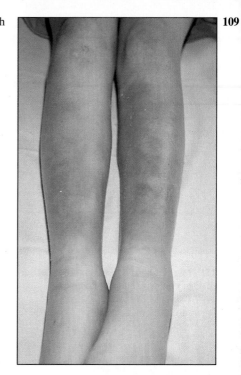

110 Ear lobe lesion in a child from Sierra Leone.
(a) What is it?
(b) Why do such lesions occur?

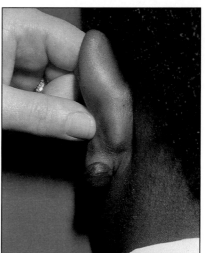

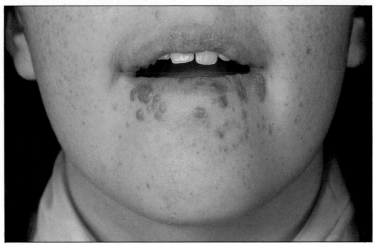

111 This 17-year-old fit young lady presented with chin papules only.
(a) Can you suggest a diagnosis?
(b) What would a skin biopsy show?
(c) In children this condition is rare and tends to present with acute symptoms. Name some.

112 An uncommon entity.
(a) What is this condition?
(b) How do you describe the clinical features?
(c) What is the prognosis?

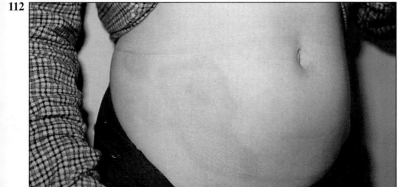

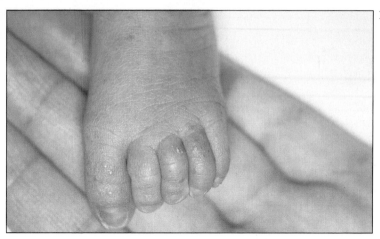

113 This benign condition, seen here on the toes, presents in neonates.
(a) What is the diagnosis?
(b) What is the natural history?

114 This lesion has a striking colour.
(a) What is it?
(b) Of what does it consist?

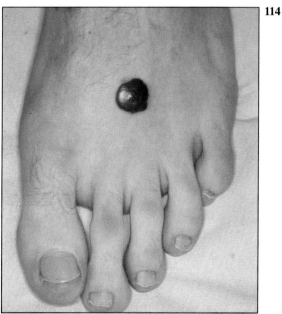

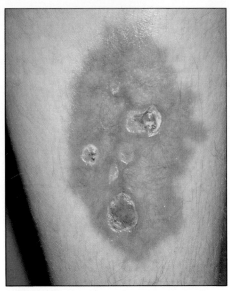

115 Lesion over left shin.
(a) What is the diagnosis?
(b) This girl has a systemic condition. What is it likely to be?
(c) What is the incidence of (a) in (b)?

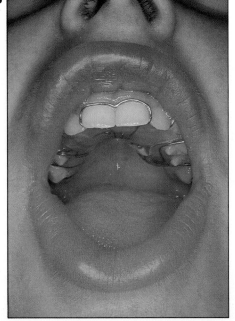

116 This child has chronic lip swelling.
(a) What do you think is the cause?
(b) What are other possible causes?

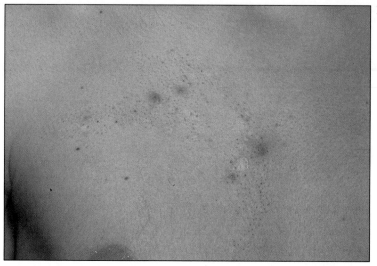

117 This lesion was localised to the chest.
(a) What is it called?
(b) Does it disappear?

118 You will see
this quite often
if you look for
it.
(a) What is it?
(b) Are there
any symptoms?
(c) What are the
features?

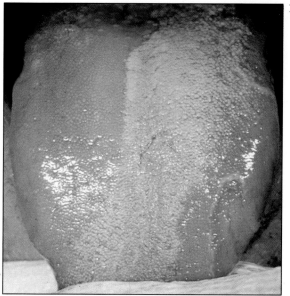

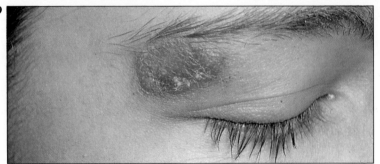

119 This lesion appeared some time after returning from a Mediterranean holiday.
(a) Do you know the diagnosis?
(b) How is it caused?
(c) What is the incubation period?
(d) What is the management?

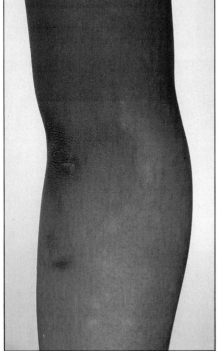

120 This condition was quite widespread.
(a) What is it?
(b) What are the features?
(c) What is the pathology?

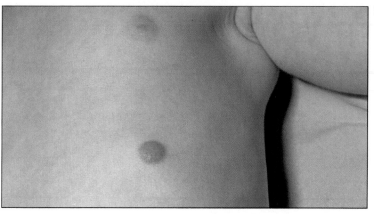

121 This lesion in a 4-month-old child has a tendency to disappear spontaneously.
(a) What is it called?
(b) Are there any associations?

122 These pigmented
lesions are uncommon at
birth, but usual afterwards.
(a) What are they?
(b) Are they benign?

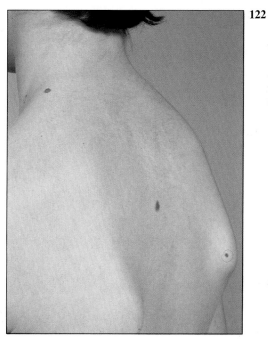

123 This child has a viral exanthem.
(a) What is the diagnosis?
(b) What is the virus?
(c) How long does the rash last?

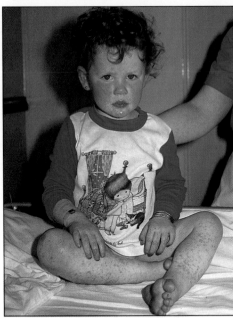

Fifth
DISEASE

124 A sign of summer.
(a) What has this child got?
(b) What is the histology?

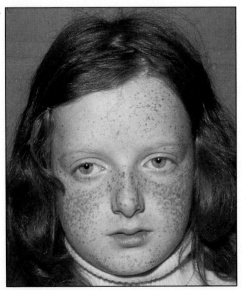

125 This Somalian child had an 18-month history of patchy scalp hair loss.
(a) What is the diagnosis?
(b) How was it confirmed?
(c) What is the treatment?

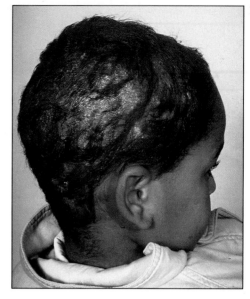

126 This condition is still seen in colder weather in homes lacking central heating.
(a) What is the little toe lesion?
(b) How do such lesions present?

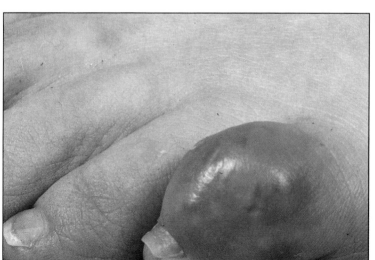

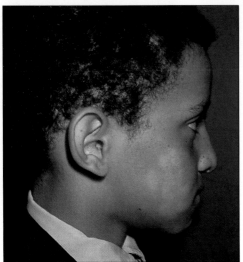

127 This condition is relatively common.
(a) What is it called?
(b) What are the features?

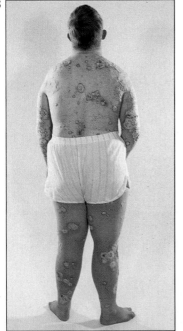

128 A common chronic genodermatosis.
(a) What is it called?
(b) What is the management?

129 This Caucasian girl has interesting hair.
(a) What is this called?
(b) What is the mode of inheritance?

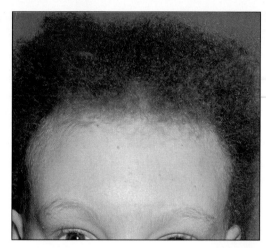

130 A 6-year-old receiving penicillin presented with a rash.
(a) How would you describe this drug-induced eruption?
(b) What advice would you give to the parents?

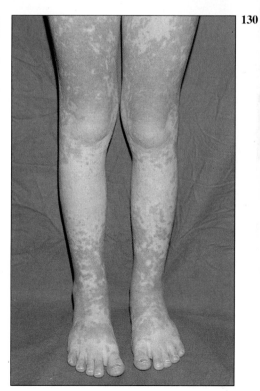

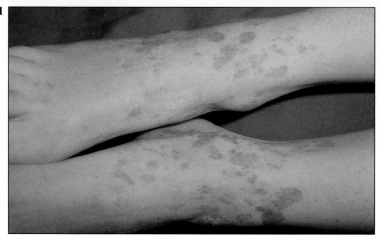

131 This is a rather chronic, often static, eruption.
(a) What is it called?
(b) What are the clinical features?
(c) What is its histopathology?

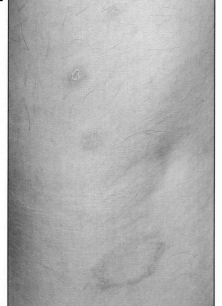

132 A presumed viral infection.
(a) What is it called?
(b) How is a first lesion often described?
(c) How long does the condition last?

133 This young girl developed a papular excoriated eruption with light exposure.
(a) What is the diagnosis?
(b) How is it managed?

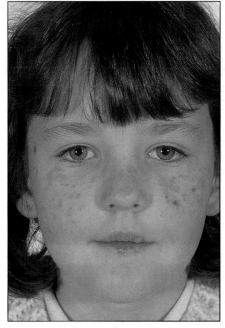

134 This boy has a well-defined acute blistering eruption.
(a) What is it?
(b) How would you treat it?

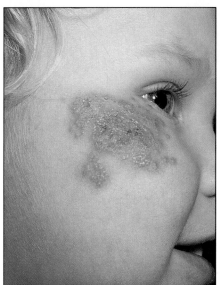

135

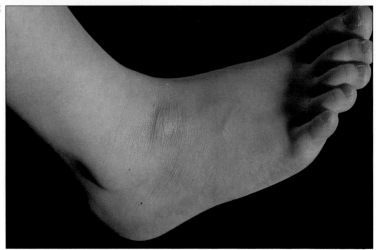

135 Not usually recognised, but relatively common.
(a) What is the diagnosis?
(b) Is treatment required?

136

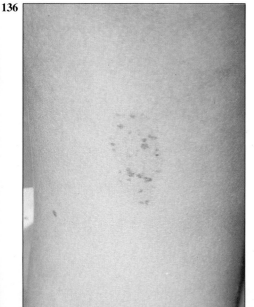

136 A well-defined patch with pigmented areas within.
(a) What is this uncommon lesion called?
(b) Is treatment necessary?

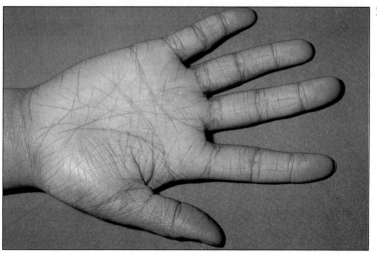

137 This child has increased palmar markings.
(a) What condition does this suggest in a child?
(b) How would you confirm the underlying disorder?

138 This is an odd, relatively common condition.
(a) What is it called?
(b) What is the natural history?

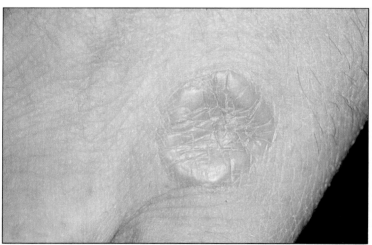

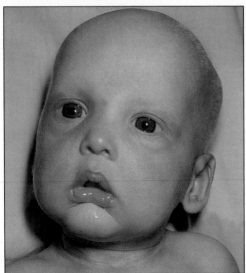

139, 140 The neonate shown has a small chin and wrinkled periorbital skin; the 3-year-old boy has the same condition.
(a) What is the diagnosis?
(b) What are some important features?
(c) How may it present acutely?

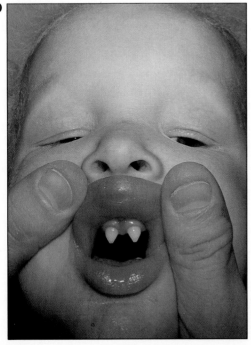

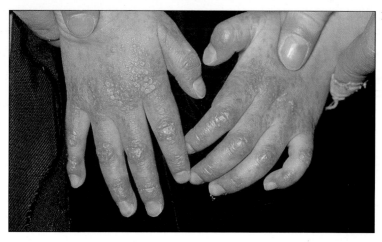

141 This little girl presented with a non-irritant eruption over her face, fingers, knees, elbows, and feet.
(a) What is the diagnosis?
(b) What other features would you look for and ask about?

142 This 5-year-old boy presented with hair thinning over the sides of the anterior scalp with preservation of hair in the midline.
(a) What do you think the diagnosis is?
(b) What is the cause?
(c) How is it managed?

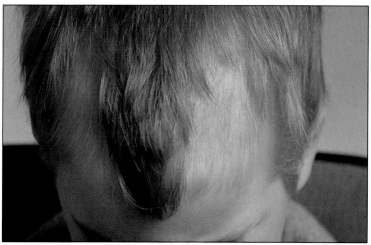

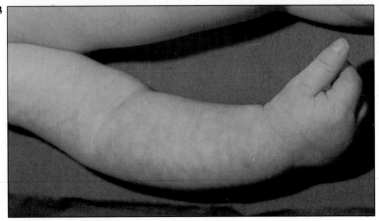

143 This is a normal finding in neonates.
(a) What is it called?
(b) Why does it occur in infants?

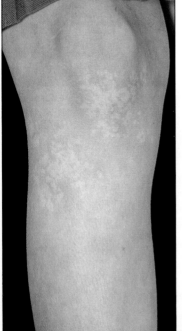

144 Persistent pale area over the knee.
(a) What is this?
(b) How can you confirm the diagnosis?

145 This is a common condition in children.
(a) What are the lesions called?
(b) What happens to them?

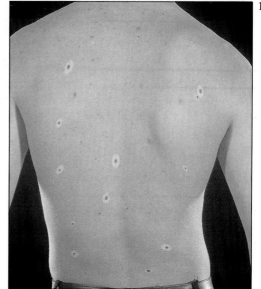

146 This is an autosomal dominant condition with skeletal, nail, and sometimes urinary tract abnormalities.
(a) What is it called?
(b) What urinary tract abnormalities?

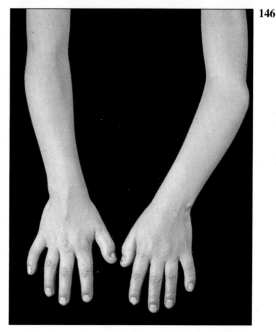

81

147 A common condition in infants and young children.
(a) What is the diagnosis?
(b) What kind of virus causes it?
(c) How long is the natural history?

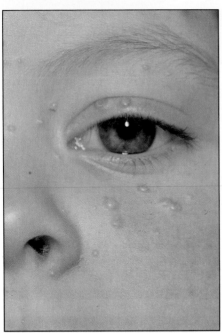

148 This irritant condition is seen most commonly in spring and summer and usually over the lower legs, at least initially.
(a) What is the diagnosis?
(b) What is the cause?

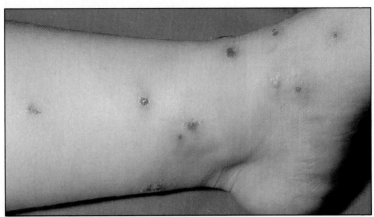

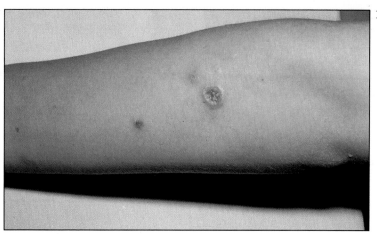

149 These are self-inflicted lesions that the patient admits producing.
(a) What is the diagnosis?
(b) How is this managed?

150 This girl has nail changes and also had a skin eruption.
(a) What do you think the diagnosis is?
(b) What will happen to the nail disorder?

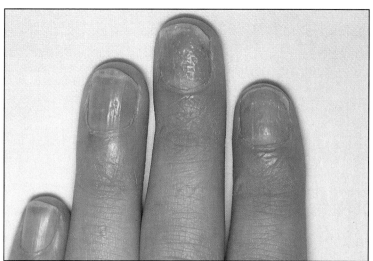

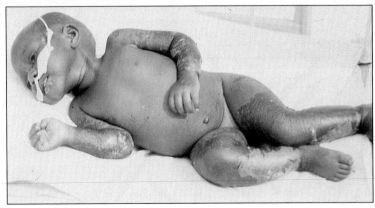

151 An 18-month-old child from Gambia.
(a) What is the diagnosis?
(b) What are the skin signs?
(c) How is this managed?

152 This solitary lesion over the left thigh urticated with rubbing.
(a) What is it called?
(b) What is the prognosis?
(c) What other types of such cell accumulations do you know?

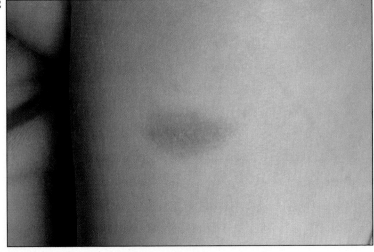

153 Rare in a child; this fit girl is only 4 years old.
(a) What is the diagnosis?
(b) What has occurred?
(c) Is the cause definitely known?

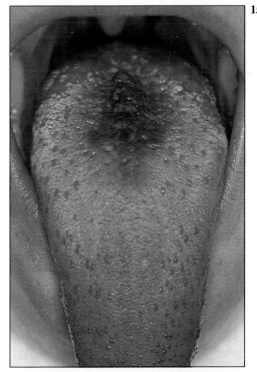

154 A common condition manifesting as a rash, particularly over buttocks and lower limbs.
(a) What is the diagnosis?
(b) What is its pathology?
(c) What are the clinical features?
(d) Comment on renal involvement.

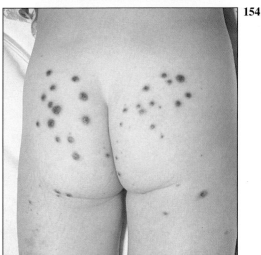

155 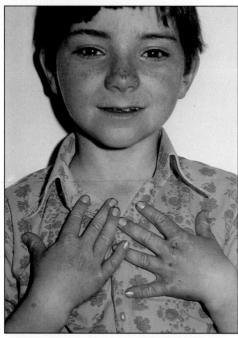 This boy developed symptoms with sun exposure before two years of age.
(a) What is the diagnosis?
(b) What are the clinical features?
(c) How can the diagnosis be confirmed?
(d) What is the treatment?

156 This 7-month-old boy presented with drowsiness and purpuric skin eruption.
(a) What is the diagnosis?
(b) What investigations would you do to confirm the diagnosis?
(c) What is the treatment?

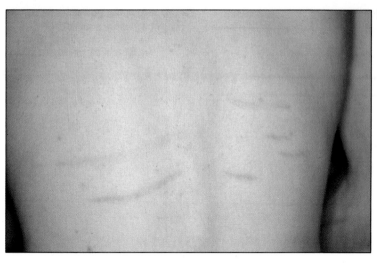

157 This is a fit young man.
(a) What are these lesions?
(b) What is their incidence?

158 A condition that is very common in primary schoolchildren.
(a) What is the diagnosis?
(b) What are the symptoms of affected individuals?

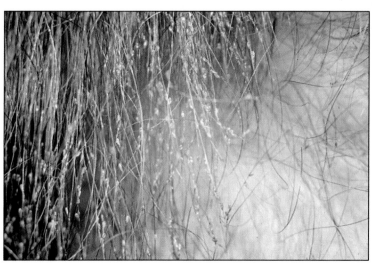

159

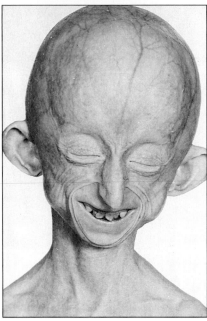

159 A rare disorder.
(a) What is it called?
(b) What are its clinical features?
(c) What is the prognosis?

160 This condition caused discomfort.
(a) What is it?
(b) What is the treatment?

160

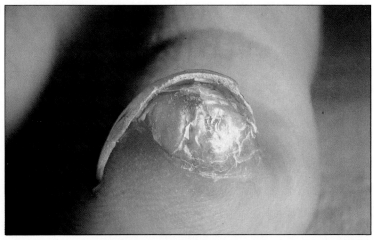

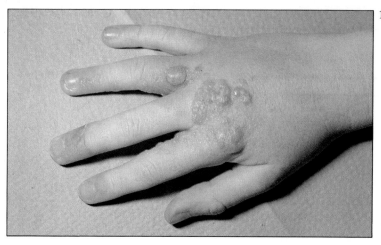

161 This boy developed a fingertip eruption under an adhesive plaster and then more plaster was applied over the back of the hand.
(a) What is the problem?
(b) How can you confirm the diagnosis?

162 This infant's napkin area eruption failed to respond to simple measures.
(a) What is the diagnosis?
(b) What investigations would you do?
(c) How would you manage this?

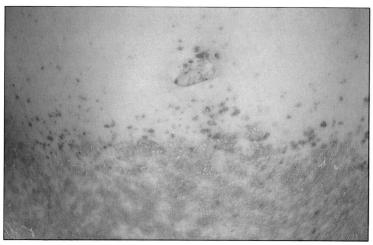

163 This baby is less than 24 hours old.
(a) What is the condition?
(b) What will happen next?

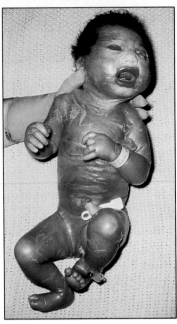

164 This 11-month-old boy has a rare vascular developmental disorder.
(a) What is it called?
(b) What is the pathology?
(c) What is the natural history?

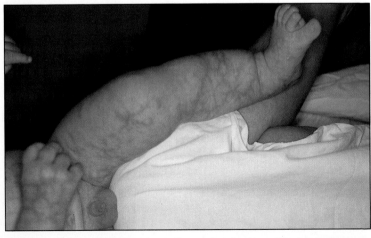

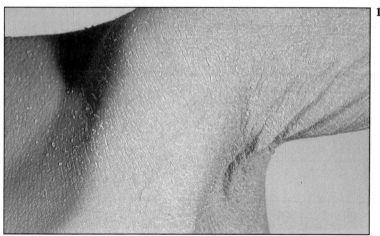

165

165, 166 Photographs taken at 4 and 6 years of age. Like her elder sister this girl was a collodion baby.
(a) What is the diagnosis?
(b) How do you treat it?

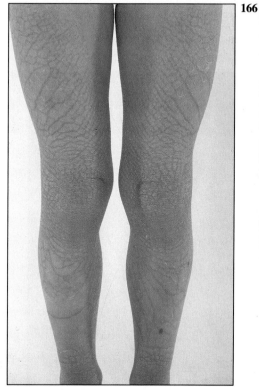
166

167

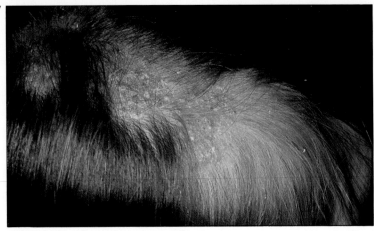

167 This girl has scalp ringworm. Her dog also had ringworm (due to *Microsporum canis*).
(a) What is this inflammatory scalp lesion called?
(b) How would you describe the appearance?

168

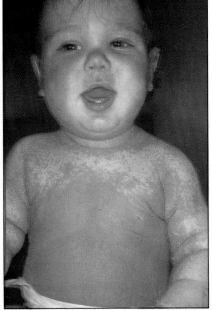

168 An uncommon condition.
(a) What is the diagnosis?
(b) What is the natural history?
(c) How would you treat it?

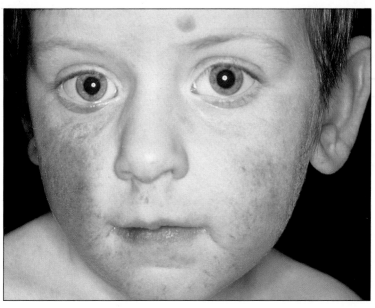

169, 170 This girl also has patches of scarring alopecia.
(a) What is the diagnosis?
(b) How is it inherited?

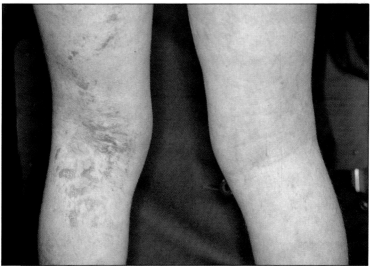

171

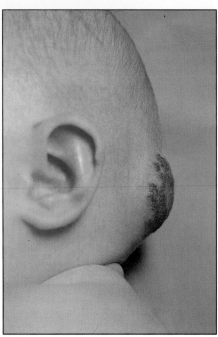

171 A common condition in infants.
(a) What is this lesion?
(b) What is the natural history?

172 A tender toe.
(a) What is the disorder of the big toenail?
(b) What is the treatment?

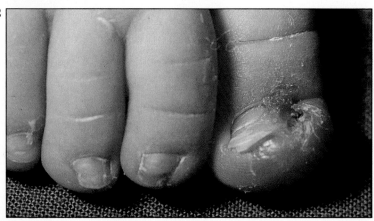

173 Grouped papules over the left shoulder, but they were more widespread.
(a) What is the diagnosis?
(b) How long does it last?

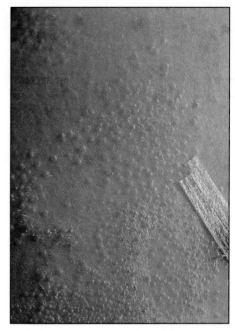

174 An irritant disorder of unknown cause occurring in infants.
(a) What is it called?
(b) Is there any treatment?

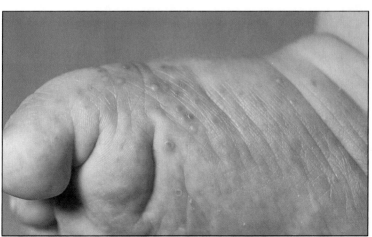

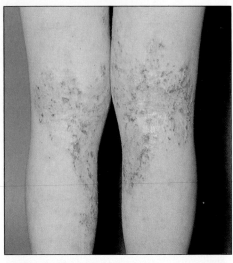

175 An irritant common everyday problem in dermatology clinics.
(a) What is the diagnosis?
(b) What is your treatment?

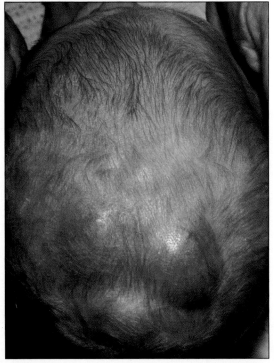

176 These huge purplish lesions were present at birth in this neonate and fluctuated in size.
(a) What is the diagnosis?
(b) What is the prognosis?

177 An infant with swollen lower limbs.

(a) What is this?

(b) What would you look for if the patient was female and had hypoplastic nails?

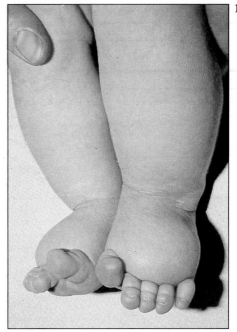

178 This is uncommon in children, but this boy is only 12 years old.

(a) What is the diagnosis?

(b) What is the treatment?

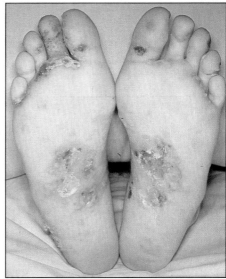

179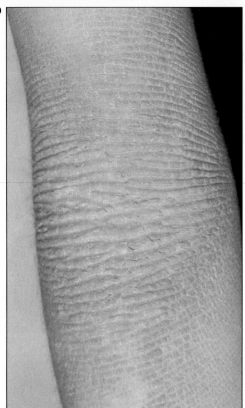

179 This 4-year-old boy was born with this condition, which is dominantly inherited.
(a) What is it called?
(b) What are the signs?
(c) How is it treated?

180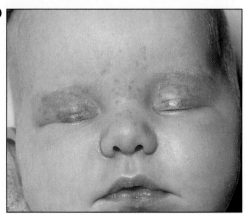

180 These are common lesions in infants.
(a) What are they called?
(b) What is the prognosis?

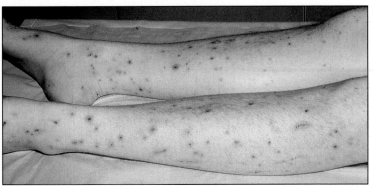

181 This 14-year-old presented with irritant skin lesions over the limbs. She also had significant weight loss, lymphadenopathy, and hypergammaglobulinaemia, and a chest radiograph revealed an anterior mediastinal mass.
(a) What is the probable diagnosis?
(b) What is the treatment?

182 This unilateral eruption cleared in a few months.
(a) What is it called?
(b) What is the histology?

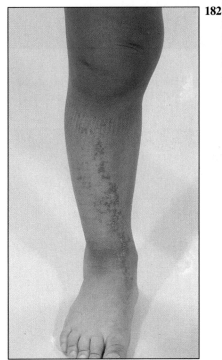

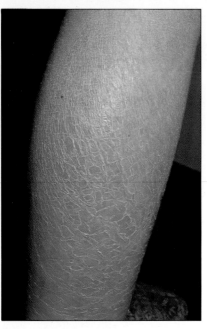

183 There are many types of this inherited condition, but this is the most common.
(a) What is the diagnosis?
(b) What are the clinical features?

184 This is a perioral eruption in a 2-year-old child.
(a) What is the diagnosis?
(b) Do you know the cause?

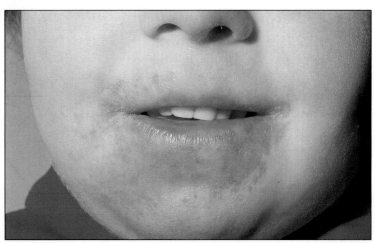

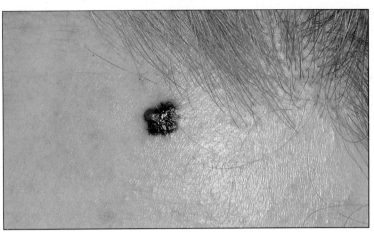

185 This boy of 17 years of age presented with this black forehead lesion, which he had had for one year.
(a) What is it?
(b) What is the treatment?

186 These were first noticed one morning on waking.
(a) What has this child got?
(b) How would you manage this?

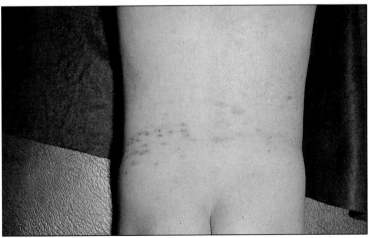

187

187 This 8-year-old boy had asymptomatic yellow plaques over his abdomen.
(a) What is this benign condition?
(b) Can such lesions occur alone?

188

188 This lesion was visible following varicella and separation of a scab below the knee.
(a) What is it called?
(b) What is the cause?
(c) How would you treat it?

189 A 4-month-old infant
with a common sign.
(a) What is the diagnosis?
(b) Why does it occur?
(c) What is the prognosis?

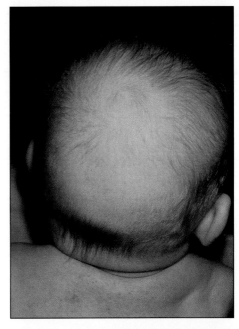

190 A 12-year-old girl with a
personal and family history of
episodes of subcutaneous
swelling affecting the face
and elsewhere, occurring
spontaneously or with
trauma, and usually requiring
no treatment. She was admitted urgently with facial
swelling following a slight
facial scratch and the
swelling became complicated
by laryngeal oedema.
(a) What is this rare disorder?
(b) What is its mode of
inheritance?
(c) What is the defect?
(d) How would you treat a
severe acute attack?

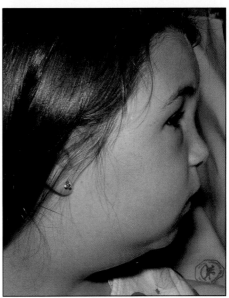

191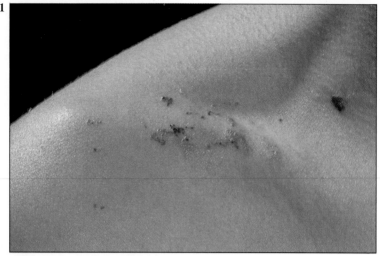

191, 192 This 14-year-old boy has a long-standing area of vesicles, some of which were haemorrhagic, over the right shoulder.
(a) Name this entity.
(b) When do the lesions usually appear?
(c) What is the routine management?

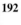

192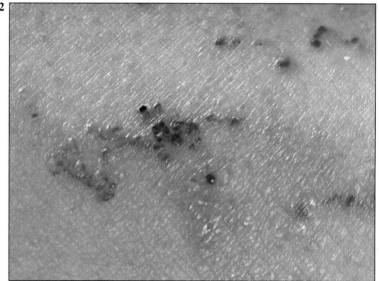

ANSWERS

1 (a) Peutz–Jeghers syndrome. Lentigines are visible around the lips.
(b) The syndrome includes oral and facial pigmentation and there may be pigmented macules over hands and feet, with polyposis of the small and large bowel.
(c) Intestinal obstruction due to intussusception.

2 (a) Candidosis.
(b) Satellite pustules indicate the diagnosis and it is likely that this was the primary disorder rather than *Candida* complicating another napkin area eruption.
(c) Oral and topical nystatin or an imidazole.

3, 4 (a) Tuberous sclerosis. Angiofibromas are visible over the face and a solitary shagreen patch over the back.
(b) Hypomelanotic macules over trunk and limbs are an early sign as is a smooth red or yellow forehead plaque. Periungual fibromas usually appear after puberty.
(c) Autosomal dominant.

5 Alopecia areata.
(b) Unknown cause, but it is likely that an immune mechanism is involved.
(c) On the whole the prognosis is directly proportional to the extent of the loss. If one or two small patches are present regrowth occurs in 6–12 months in 80% of individuals. The prognosis tends to be poor when associated with atopy. The condition can sometimes recur.

6 (a) Erythema multiforme.
(b) Target lesions.
(c) Well-known recognised causes are herpes simplex, mycoplasma infection, and drugs, including penicillin and sulphonamides.
(d) Erythema multiforme can be separated into minor and major forms and the severe major form is termed Stevens-Johnson syndrome.

7 (a) Atopic dermatitis.
(b) Mildly potent topical corticosteroid combined with antiseptic or antibiotic, emollients, and an oral antihistamine.
(c) On the whole the condition improves with increasing age. Up to 65% of children are clear by 11 years of age, and many clear earlier.

8 (a) Cellulitis.
(b) Streptococcal infection entering through a scratch/sore over the face.
(c) Intramuscular benzylpenicillin for the first 24 hours and then oral phenoxymethylpenicillin for a week.

9 (a) Scalp cyst. This was in fact a rather rare entity showing glial cell heteropia.
(b) Leptomeningeal cyst, cephalocele, vascular naevi.
(c) Excision.

10 (a) Capillary haemangioma (strawberry mark).
(b) Growth for about a year, followed by resolution, often complete, within 4–5 years.
(c) Observation only, generally. Lesions that grow rapidly or appear around vital areas (eyes, throat) may merit short-term systemic corticosteroid therapy to encourage involution. Surgery including laser therapy may occasionally be indicated for corticosteroid-resistant lesions.

11 (a) Ringworm (tinea unguium).

(b) By culture of toenail clippings after direct examination of scrapings in a potassium hydroxide preparation.

(c) Oral griseofulvin 10 mg/kilogram body weight daily.

12 (a) Lichen sclerosus et atrophicus.

(b) Eroded skin with white edge to lesions.

(c) Varies. Potent topical corticosteroids may be necessary in the short term but some patients are asymptomatic and prefer simple emollients.

(d) Guarded, but many clear before puberty.

13 (a) Urticaria.

(b) Ordinary (non-physical) urticaria has many causes. Acute urticaria may be due to drugs, food, or inhalants, but in many patients no cause is found.

(c) Antihistamines. Intravenous hydrocortisone may be necessary in severe acute attacks with angioedema, or intramuscular adrenaline 0.05–0.5 ml depending on age, of 1 in 1000 (1 mg/ml).

14 (a) Hand, foot and mouth disease.

(b) Vesicles with surrounding erythema. Lesions may affect palms, mouth, and buttocks.

(c) Coxsackie viruses type A16, A10, A5.

(d) Minor illness, usually resolving in about a week.

15 (a) Ashy dermatosis (erythema dyschromicum perstans).

(b) Unknown.

16 (a) Herpes simplex (primary infection).

(b) Ulcerated tongue and lips.

(c) Soft food and drink for a few days and topical antiseptic/antibiotic if skin lesions become secondarily infected.

17 (a) Infantile gluteal granuloma.

(b) Nodules over the vulva.

(c) Usually there is a background of irritant napkin dermatitis and the granulomas follow overuse of, often potent, topical corticosteroids, for this.

18 (a) Mongolian patches.

(b) They indicate the presence of spindle-shaped melanocytes in the dermis.

(c) Slow resolution but may take many years to disappear.

19, 20 (a) BCG (Bacillus Calmette–Guérin).

(b) Ulceration, probably following an injection that was too deep. Ulcers usually heal spontaneously, but cleaning with saline soaks and 3% chlortetracycline ointment or cream may be helpful.

(c) BCG lupus. There is usually spontaneous healing, but the above treatment and/or erythromycin 1 g daily for 2–4 weeks is usually curative.

21 (a) Perianal dermatitis.

(b) Diarrhoea, antibiotic therapy, threadworms. Streptococcal infection may complicate dermatitis.

(c) Depends on the cause, but should be sought and not assumed.

22 (a) Diffuse neonatal haemangiomatosis. Diffuse indicating multiple organ involvement.
(b) Poor, as in this infant who died when 2 months old. Interferon α–2a may have a place in treatment.

23 (a) Guttate psoriasis.
(b) An attack commonly persists for a few months and is often followed by a prolonged remission.
(c) Bland applications because of the tendency to spontaneous resolution.

24 (a) Pachyonychia congenita.
(b) Autosomal dominant.
(c) Abnormal nails at birth, which develop wedge-like thickening with exaggeration of the transverse curvature. Palmar and plantar hyperkeratosis. Oral leukoplakia frequently occurs in later childhood.

25 (a) Vitiligo. The trunk is illustrated.
(b) Melanocytes are destroyed.
(c) Unsatisfactory. It is important to protect affected areas from the sun with adequate topical sunscreen preparations.

26 (a) Immune thrombocytopenic purpura. Often occurs after a viral infection, particularly rubella.
(b) The majority recover spontaneously within a few months.

27, 28 (a) Staphylococcal scalded skin syndrome.
(b) Production of an exotoxin from phage Group 2 benzylpenicillin-resistant staphylococci.
(c) Penicillinase-resistant penicillin such as flucloxacillin or fucidic acid.

29 (a) Scleroedema.
(b) Unknown. A preceding infection is quite common.
(c) Usually begins over back, neck or face with symmetrical tightness of the skin and loss of facial expression.
(d) Tends to resolve within two years.

30 (a) Varicella. Rather haemorrhagic in this boy.
(b) 14–21 days.
(c) Until scales separate following crusting of vesicles.

31 (a) Irritant napkin dermatitis.
(b) Pressure/friction at sites of napkin contact with skin.
(c) Exposure if practical. Simple emollients and a mildly potent corticosteroid are indicated.

32 (a) Scabies. Burrow visible over heel.
(b) Yes. Those in close contact are likely to be affected.
(c) A single application below the face of lindane 1% lotion, without a preceding bath, to all areas and left on for 8–12 hours. Alternatively 25% benzyl benzoate emulsion applied similarly but left on for 24 hours and repeated once only: it is irritant and should be applied in 1/3 strength to infants and 1/2 strength to children. Other scabicides are malathion (0.5%) and permethrin (5%).

33 (a) Infantile acne. This appears between the age of 3 months and 5 years.

(b) In the great majority of cases there is no evidence of endocrine disorder.

(c) Topical applications and sometimes oral erythromycin. Oral tetracyclines should be avoided in children up to 12 years of age of in view of the possibility of unsightly teeth staining.

34 (a) Beau's lines.

(b) Temporary interruption of nail formation associated with severe illness or shock.

35, 36, 37 (a) Epidermolysis bullosa.

(b) There are three principal types (simplex, dystrophic, junctional), but there are numerous subtypes. The first picture shows a 19-day-old boy with blistering from birth. He has epidermolysis bullosa (e.b.) simplex (Dowling–Meara type) and improved with increasing age. The feet are of a girl who developed blisters limited to hands and feet as a teenager: she has e.b. simplex (Weber–Cockayne). The brothers have a more severe scarring e.b. of dominant dystrophic type.

(c) In the simplex forms the plane of separation is through the epidermis, but it is below this in the other more severe forms.

(d) Protection of the skin from mechanical trauma.

38 (a) Supernumerary nipple.

(b) Along the course of the embryological milk lines which run from the anterior axillary folds to the inner thighs.

39 (a) Urticaria pigmentosa.

(b) Multiple pigmented papules over the trunk some of which are urticated.

(c) Antihistamines if itching/flushing is marked. Oral sodium cromoglycate, which blocks mast cell degranulation, is also useful.

(d) Resolution is usual in children, but may take years.

40 (a) Malalignment of the big toe nail. May involve one or both big toes.

(b) Spontaneous resolution may occur but marked deviation can be treated by surgery with realignment of the whole nail apparatus, but this should be carried out before 2 years of age.

41 (a) Faun-tail naevus.

(b) Full neurological examination is indicated because of the possible association of spinal cord abnormalities with an underlying spina bifida.

42 (a) Bitten nails (onychophagia).

(b) Anxiety, tension or stress may play a part. It is an extremely common habit. Up to 33% of children between the ages of 7 and 10 are nail biters.

43, 44 (a) Gianotti–Crosti syndrome (papular acrodermatitis).

(b) Coppery red non-itchy papules which appear over face, extremities, and buttocks, but spare the trunk.

(c) The disorder is probably viral in origin and hepatitis B antigen has been reported in some cases. Coxsackie, Epstein–Barr, and parainfluenza viruses may also be responsible.

(d) Self-limiting, tending to last weeks.

45 (a) Spindle-cell naevus (Spitz naevus, juvenile melanoma). A benign tumour.
(b) No. They are usually smooth-surfaced and dome-shaped, but colour can be very variable from pink to black.
(c) By histological examination of excised lesions. Cells are generally spindle-shaped and mitotic figures are also present. Kamino bodies (eosinophilic globules) in the epidermis are usual.

46 (a) Intertrigo. A moist flexural eruption seen particularly in overweight infants or may be a sign of infantile seborrhoeic dermatitis.
(b) A cream containing an antibacterial in combination with a mild corticosteroid is helpful.

47 (a) Angioma serpiginosum. This is a rare disorder of upper dermal capillaries and venules, which show localised dilatations. Onset is usually in childhood.
(b) Individual puncta may disappear, but complete resolution is uncommon.

48 (a) Diabetes mellitus.
(b) Yes, following control of her insulin-dependent disorder.

49 (a) Acrodermatitis enteropathica. An autosomal recessive condition seen particularly in infants at the time of weaning or earlier in bottle fed infants.
(b) It is thought to be due to a defect in the absorption of zinc from the bowel.
(c) Oral zinc sulphate.
(d) Acquired zinc deficiency can result from an inadequate dietary intake, increased zinc loss or intravenous nutrition. Even in the breast fed infant, low zinc levels may precipitate a zinc deficiency. Remember that premature infants are in negative zinc balance.

50 (a) Perianal warts.
(b) By transmission of virus from another site or other person.
(c) Liquid nitrogen, low concentration podophyllin, and occasionally surgery for extensive unresponsive lesions.

51 (a) Dermatitis artefacta.
(b) The bizarre nature of the lesions gives a clue and an unconcerned attitude will support suspicion.
(c) Affected individuals tend to be female, adolescent, intellectually dull, and unsophisticated. They may be attention-seeking or self-mutilating as a protest.

52 (a) Non-accidental injury affecting the face. Bruising and swelling are visible.
(b) The child should be fully examined with a nurse and preferably a parent also present. Relevant findings should be documented with drawings/photographs. The child should generally be admitted under a Consultant Paediatrician experienced in child abuse.

53 (a) Uncombable hair. Hair shafts are abnormal in this condition.
(b) Usually around the age of 3 years scalp hair becomes disorderly and remains so despite brushing and combing.
(c) Spontaneous improvement tends to occur.

54 (a) Dermographism (factitious urticaria). A physical urticaria.
(b) A wealing tendency with light trauma, which can be observed in 5% of normal people and which may or may not be symptomatic (i.e. presenting with itching).

55 (a) Congenital giant pigmented naevus. These are melanocytic naevi presenting as extensive (> 20 cm in diameter) pigmented hairy areas.

(b) Early surgical excision wherever possible because of the 6% risk of malignant change, which is most common in the first decade.

56 (a) Wiskott–Aldrich syndrome.

(b) X-linked recessive.

(c) Poor, unless the condition is treated by bone marrow transplantation.

57 (a) Measles.

(b) Bronchopneumonia, otitis media.

58 (a) Subungual haemorrhage. This resulted from wearing platform shoes.

(b) Use of more suitable footwear.

59 (a) Raynaud's syndrome.

(b) A typical attack consists of pallor in one or more fingers, followed by cyanosis and then erythema.

(c) There may be no apparent cause, as in this girl, who was followed up for many years. However, Raynaud's syndrome may be secondary to systemic sclerosis, or other conditions such as occlusive arterial disease, or a cervical rib.

60 (a) Scabies.

(b) 2–6 weeks.

(c) By demonstrating mites, egg, or mite faeces in scrapings from lesions. A positive history of contacts would also be useful evidence.

61 (a) Gum hypertrophy.

(b) Cyclosporin as in this child, but also phenytoin.

62 (a) Incontinentia pigmenti (Bloch–Sulzberger syndrome).

(b) Linear or grouped vesicles appear over trunk and limbs, but by the end of the first month small firm papules and warty plaques appear. These leave angulated and streaked pigmentation and there may be hypopigmentation.

(c) Dental, skeletal, eye, and central nervous system abnormalities may occur.

63 (a) Lip licking.

(b) The habit is more common in atopics.

64 (a) Chronic paronychia.

(b) It is seen most commonly in thumb/finger suckers/biters. A mixed flora of bacteria and *Candida albicans* is often found.

65 (a) Pityriasis amiantacea.

(b) May occur as an isolated abnormality or as a sign of psoriasis or seborrhoeic dermatitis.

(c) A tar/salicylic acid-containing ointment is useful.

66 (a) Inflamed linear epidermal naevus.

(b) Appearance in infancy and usually a female. It is itchy, linear, and usually unilateral over lower limb and buttock.

67 (a) Jelly fish sting.
(b) Pouring vinegar onto the area of the sting and removing any attached tentacles as quickly as possible. Cold packs also provide relief.

68 (a) Ehlers–Danlos syndrome.
(b) There are ten clinically and genetically distinct varieties all associated with abnormalities of collagen.
(c) The most common types (I. II, III) are inherited in an autosomal dominant manner.

69 (a) Callosities.
(b) He had the habit of biting his skin.

70 (a) Sebaceous naevus.
(b) Benign or malignant transformation particularly basal cell carcinoma is not uncommon and usually occurs from the fourth decade.
(c) Excision in adolescence or early adult life as a precaution.

71 (a) Chronic bullous disease of childhood (linear IgA dermatosis of childhood).
(b) Usually before 6 years of age. Tense bullae over lower trunk, genitalia, and lower limbs; blisters often occur in ringed patterns. Conjunctival scarring may occur.
(c) Dapsone may be helpful, but use has to be carefully monitored.
(d) This rare condition may clear spontaneously within 2–3 years.

72 (a) Systemic sclerosis. Binding down of the skin and restricted movement of fingers is shown.
(b) Regular assessment of pulmonary, bowel, and renal function is important. Treatment is unsatisfactory and nonspecific.

73 (a) Impetigo.
(b) It is usually due to *Staphylococcus aureus,* but may be complicated by streptococcus.
(c) Removal of crusts is essential and then antiseptic/antibiotic ointment should be applied. If widespread and/or haemolytic streptococci are present, oral antibiotic therapy is indicated; this may help prevent the occasional complication of acute glomerulonephritis following streptococcal impetigo.

74 (a) Erythrokeratoderma.
(b) Symmetrical persistent hyperkeratotic hyperpigmented patches. There may also be a migrating erythematous eruption in one form of the condition.

75 (a) Contact dermatitis. Nickel allergy.
(b) Patch testing with standard concentrations of various chemicals to detect epidermal sensitivity.

76 (a) Calcinosis cutis. Localised to the finger and of unknown cause in this boy.
(b) May be secondary to metabolic disorders or to tissue damage in connective tissue disorders.

77 (a) Miliaria. Caused by eccrine sweat retention.
(b) Therapy is directed towards avoidance of excessive heat and humidity, with lightweight loose clothing recommended.

78 (a) Juvenile plantar dermatosis.
(b) Over the flexor aspect of the big toes.
(c) Synthetic footwear with little or absent permeability and poor moisture absorption is important.

79 (a) Portwine stain (naevus flammeus).
(b) Cosmetic cover is still the routine treatment, but laser therapy is becoming more widely available.
(c) A syndrome characterised by a portwine stain in the distribution of the first branch of the trigeminal nerve associated with a vascular malformation of the ipsilateral meninges and cerebral cortex.

80 (a) Xeroderma pigmentosum. This boy has a squamous carcinoma involving his upper lip and another had already invaded his right orbit.
(b) It is rare and characterised by hypersensitivity to ultraviolet light followed eventually by development of multiple tumours in the exposed areas.
(c) A defect of the normal repair mechanism of DNA damaged by ultraviolet rays.
(d) Protection from sunlight exposure is paramount.

81 (a) Eczema herpeticum. Usually a primary herpes simplex infection and complicating atopic dermatitis in this child.
(b) Acyclovir, an antiviral agent, is the treatment indicated in severe cases: there are both topical and systemic preparations.

82 (a) Pyogenic granuloma (granuloma telangiectaticum).
(b) It is a rapidly developing vascular nodule, which often occurs at a site of recent injury particularly over a finger.
(c) Curettage followed by diathermy coagulation of the base.

83, 84 (a) Pityriasis lichenoides. Close-up shows a characteristic crumb-like scale.
(b) Reddish-brown, slightly raised papules with lesions most marked over trunk. Some lesions are haemorrhagic, some necrotic and others show the scale.
(c) May last months or years but tends to be months in children.

85 (a) Keratosis pilaris. The term describes a horny plugging of follicles.
(b) It usually affects backs of upper arms and front of thighs and is common.

86 (a) Tylosis (tylosis palmaris et plantaris).
(b) Autosomal dominant.
(c) No. It is usually benign, but a rare association between tylosis appearing in childhood rather than infancy, oral preleukoplakia and/or leukoplakia in tylotic children and adults, and the development of oesophageal carcinoma in adult life, has been described in two Liverpool families.

87 (a) Warty epidermal naevus (localised).
(b) It presents at birth or in infancy, often growing with the individual until late adolescence.
(c) Can be left alone. However, if requiring treatment, excision is recommended. Cryotherapy or cautery will be followed by recurrence sooner or later.

88 (a) Oculocutaneous albinism.

(b) Autosomal recessive.

(c) Two. Tyrosinase-negative and tyrosinase-positive. From a clinical point of view some pigment is found in the positive type and the patient may have the ability to tan. This baby was considered tyrosinase-negative.

(d) Restriction of exposure to ultraviolet light and use of a high (>15) sun protection factor (SPF) sunscreen are essential.

89, 90 (a) Acute haemorrhagic oedema of infancy. Some consider this rare condition a variant of Henoch–Schönlein purpura, but it is probably a distinct entity.

(b) Infants between 4 months and 2 years.

(c) Inflammatory oedema and purpura on the limbs and face. Lesions over limbs are often medallion-like. Visceral involvement is very uncommon.

(d) Spontaneous resolution occurs within 1–3 weeks.

91, 92 (a) Aplasia cutis. A rare developmental deformity.

(b) Most common over the vertex of the scalp in or adjacent to the midline as one or more well-defined non-inflammatory oval or circular ulcers, crusted areas, or scars.

(c) These include secondary infection, bleeding, and meningitis with deeper lesions.

(d) Most lesions are superficial and heal within a few weeks. Larger defects, like the one illustrated, require protection (he wore a rubber helmet) and later may undergo scar excision and use of tissue expanders before closing the defect.

93 (a) Von–Recklinghausen neurofibromatosis (NF-1).

(b) Café au lait patches, which usually develop within the first year of life and may be present at birth; there may also be bilateral axillary and inguinal freckling; cutaneous neurofibromas, which do not develop until later childhood; iris hamartomas (Lisch nodules) develop in time in all patients. Congenital bone anomalies and peripheral nerve and CNS tumours (particularly optic glioma) occur.

94 (a) Neonatal lupus erythematosus.

(b) Discoid scaling erythematous lesions, particularly over the face. There is an increased incidence of congenital heart block.

(c) Both mother and child are usually positive for the anti-RO/SSA antibody and generally show a speckled pattern of fluorescent antinuclear antibodies.

95 (a) Black heel (talon noir). An asymptomatic condition, which tends to be bilateral, in athletic adolescents.

(b) Papillary dermal capillaries are ruptured by the shearing action associated with the particular sport.

96 (a) Viral warts.

(b) A DNA-containing papillomavirus.

(c) In children virtually all disappear spontaneously within 3 years and may disappear in months.

97 (a) Sex-linked ichthyosis.

(b) Steroid sulphatase deficiency is common. Its absence permits identification of maternal carriers.

(c) Urea-containing emollient creams are helpful.

98 (a) 20-nail dystrophy.
(b) Alopecia areata and lichen planus are causes, but most cases are of unknown cause.
(c) Tends to be self-limiting and reversible, but severe individual nail damage will persist.

99 (a) Spider naevus (spider telangiectasia).
(b) Yes.
(c) In the older child, cautery or diathermy to the central arteriole.

100 (a) Herpes zoster (affecting the left trigeminal nerve).
(b) A severe attack merits systemic acyclovir.

101, 102 (a) Infantile seborrhoeic dermatitis.
(b) Appearance within the first few months of life. Napkin area, axillae, neck and post-auricular areas are usually affected. Yellowish greasy scalp is usual (cradle cap). Candida is a common secondary invader in the napkin area.
(c) Yes, but it is more often part of a widespread eruption.

103 (a) Bullous impetigo. A staphylococcal infection.
(b) A penicillinase-resistant penicillin or fusidic acid.

104 (a) Sunburn (acute solar dermatitis).
(b) Calamine lotion and mildly potent topical corticosteroids in severe acute cases. Proper preventive measures are most important, particularly for infants and fairskinned individuals.

105 (a) Acne vulgaris (common adolescent acne).
(b) Blackheads (comedones), papules, pustules.
(c) Topical treatments include benzoyl peroxide and retinoic acid creams. Oral tetracyclines are the first-line oral antibiotic therapy. Soap and water are to be encouraged.

106 (a) Loose anagen syndrome.
(b) Tends to improve with time.

107 (a) Psoriasis.
(b) Tar and salicylic acid ointments to separate the thick scales and improve the condition.

108 (a) Neonatal cold injury.
(b) The child should be kept warm and spontaneous resolution leaving no permanent damage is expected within a week or so.

109 (a) Erythema nodosum.
(b) Causes include throat infections including streptococcal (a common cause), primary tuberculous infections, sarcoidosis, cat scratch fever, *Yersinia* infections, drugs. No cause is found in about 30% of patients.

110 (a) Keloid.
(b) They represent an exaggerated connective tissue response to skin injury. Black and other dark-skinned individuals are more susceptible and the tendency is often familial.

111 (a) Sarcoidosis.
(b) Characteristic non-caseating granulomatous lesions.
(c) Weight loss, low-grade fever, bone and joint pain, fatigue.

112 (a) Morphoea. The common form of cutaneous scleroderma is shown.
(b) A slowly enlarging red or purple plaque in which the skin is firm and bound down to underlying tissue.
(c) Tends to resolve spontaneously, often leaving hyperpigmentation.

113 (a) Transient neonatal pustulosis (transient neonatal pustular melanosis).
(b) This uncommon condition persists for a few weeks only.

114 (a) Blue naevus. The rare cellular type is illustrated, which is more striking than the ordinary type.
(b) Aberrant collections of functioning benign melanocytes.

115 (a) Necrobiosis lipoidica.
(b) Diabetes mellitus.
(c) 0.3%.

116 (a) Crohn's disease. This girl had thickening and folding of the buccal mucosa and gastrointestinal investigations confirmed the diagnosis of Crohn's disease.
(b) Developmental abnormalities such as lymphangioma and haemangioma, granulomatous cheilitis of unknown cause, post-traumatic.

117 (a) Comedone naevus.
(b) No. It persists and may extend locally in childhood.

118 (a) Geographic tongue (erythema migrans).
(b) Sore tongue, but it is often asymptomatic.
(c) Map-like red areas with patterns changing from day to day.

119 (a) Cutaneous leishmaniasis.
(b) Results from the bite of an infected sandfly.
(c) Incubation period following the bite varies from weeks to months.
(d) Spontaneous healing with scarring usually takes place within a year. Standard treatment of unsightly or extensive lesions is with sodium stibogluconate.

120 (a) Idiopathic guttate hypomelanosis.
(b) Porcelain white macules over sun-exposed areas of limbs and illustrated over the forearm here.
(c) Decrease in melanin pigment granules.

121 (a) Juvenile xanthogranuloma.
(b) Usually a benign isolated condition, but has been associated with neurofibromatosis and myelogenous leukaemia.

122 (a) Acquired melanocytic naevi (naevocellular naevi).
(b) Yes. Only a very small percentage become malignant, usually in adult life. Thus, alteration of such a naevus in adult life is important.

123 (a) Erythema infectiosum (fifth disease). Note the slapped cheek appearance and maculo-papular rash over the limbs.
(b) Due to human parvovirus B-19.
(c) About 10 days, but may reappear temporarily.

124 (a) Freckles (ephelides).
(b) Temporary overproduction of melanin by a normal number of melanocytes.

125 (a) Ringworm (tinea capitis). *Trichophyton violaceum* in this child.
(b) By direct examination of hairs in 30% potassium hydroxide on a slide and by culture on Sabouraud's dextrose agar.
(c) Oral griseofulvin 10 mg/kg body weight/day, usually for 6–8 weeks.

126 (a) Chilblains (perniosis).
(b) Itchy swellings, which may blister or ulcerate.

127 (a) Pityriasis alba.
(b) Occurs in children 3–16 years of age, and usually over the face. Small patches of hypopigmentation sometimes with slight scaling and erythema may precede the hypopigmentation. Many children with this condition are atopics.

128 (a) Psoriasis. Common plaque type (psoriasis vulgaris). He also happens to have Down's syndrome.
(b) Coal tar solution can be used as a bath additive. Dithranol (anthralin) is very effective in plaque psoriasis. Most individuals with chronic psoriasis find sunlight and ultraviolet B light have a beneficial effect.

129 (a) Hereditary woolly hair.
(b) Usually autosomal dominant, but sometimes autosomal recessive.

130 (a) Exanthematic drug eruption.
(b) All penicillins to be avoided in future.

131 (a) Pigmented purpuric dermatosis.
(b) Asymptomatic dark-red or brown purpuric patches with haemosiderin staining, particularly over the lower legs.
(c) Lymphocytic vasculitis with extravasation of red blood cells and haemosiderin deposition.

132 (a) Pityriasis rosea. A presumed virus infection.
(b) A 'herald' patch.
(c) 4–6 weeks.

133 (a) Actinic prurigo.
(b) Advice on suitable clothing, restriction of ultraviolet exposure, and use of sun screening agents with a high sun protection factor (SPF).

134 (a) Herpes simplex. Recurrent (secondary) infection.
(b) Topical acyclovir cream applied 5 times daily as soon as tingling starts and to intact blisters.

135 (a) Talar callosity. A common unrecognised lesion over the anterolateral aspect of the ankle, anteromedial to the lateral malleolus.
(b) Usually none.

136 (a) Naevus spilus. The histology is that of a melanocytic naevus.
(b) No.

137 (a) Atopic dermatitis and/or ichthyosis vulgaris.
(b) History and clinical examination are usually adequate.

138 (a) Granuloma annulare.
(b) Lesions tend to disappear spontaneously, without scarring.

139, 140 (a) Hypohidrotic ectodermal dysplasia.
(b) Eccrine sweat glands are absent or diminished in number and total sweating is slight. There are also absent or abnormal teeth (pointed 'tiger' teeth are illustrated) and sparse fine fair hair.
(c) Fever of obscure origin may be the only manifestation, but infection must always be sought in febrile episodes.

141 (a) Dermatomyositis.
(b) Muscle weakness of proximal limb muscles and anterior neck muscles is a common early symptom.

142 (a) Trichotillomania (self-inflicted hair pulling).
(b) Many. May just be a habit associated with boredom, or due to chronic social deprivation, or occasionally an obsessive-compulsive disorder.
(c) Depends on the cause. The prognosis in a young child is good, but guarded in adolescent females.

143 (a) Cutis marmorata.
(b) It is a physiological response to chilling and disappears with re-warming.

144 (a) Naevus anaemicus.
(b) Under diascopic pressure (using a glass microscope slide) the naevus becomes indistinguishable from the blanched surrounding skin. Rubbing lesional skin does not produce any change in the lesion.

145 (a) Halo naevus. Depigmentation surrounding a central, commonly compound, melanocytic naevus.
(b) Lesions (halo and central) have a tendency to spontaneous resolution over many years.

146 (a) Nail-patella syndrome.
(b) Renal presenting as chronic glomerulonephritis.

147 (a) Molluscum contagiosum.
(b) Pox virus.
(c) Lesions disappear spontaneously, usually within a year.

148 (a) Papular urticaria.
(b) Hypersensitivity reaction to a bite from a flea, bed bug, mosquito, or dog louse.

149 (a) Neurotic excoriations. Unlike dermatitis artefacta the patient admits causing the lesions.
(b) Mild topical corticosteroid-antibacterial applications and seek to sort out the cause of the problem.

150 (a) Psoriasis of the nails. Pitting and minor onycholysis are visible.
(b) Return to normal with time.

151 (a) Kwashiorkor. Associated with severe protein malnutrition and relative carbohydrate excess.
(b) Pitting oedema, usually of the lower limbs. Hyperpigmented scaly plaques, especially prominent on the limbs; they peel leaving hypopigmented macules.
(c) Correction of the underlying malnutrition is the main priority. Skimmed milk is most useful.

152 (a) Mast cell naevus.
(b) Good. Disappears within years.
(c) Urticaria pigmentosa, diffuse cutaneous mastocytosis (rare).

153 (a) Black hairy tongue.
(b) A rapid proliferation of filiform papillae.
(c) No. There was no history of antibiotic therapy or smoking and she was not debilitated.

154 (a) Henoch–Schönlein purpura (anaphylactoid purpura). In about one-third of patients there is a preceding upper respiratory tract infection.
(b) The histology is of a leucocytoclastic vasculitis with extravasation of red blood cells.
(c) Affected children are usually 3 or more years old. Purpura occurs predominantly over lower limbs and buttocks. Oedema of face, hands, arms, feet, and scrotum is common. Arthritis and gastrointestinal symptoms are common.
(d) When it occurs it is usually a transient microscopic haematuria, but a few patients progress to renal failure.

155 (a) Erythropoietic protoporphyria.
(b) Burning or tingling of face and hands occurs after exposure to sunlight; affected areas may develop fine scars.
(c) Transient fluorescence of red blood cells confirms the diagnosis.
(d) Oral beta-carotene is helpful in many cases.

156 (a) Meningococcaemia.
(b) Cultures should be taken from blood, cerebrospinal fluid, skin lesions.
(c) High dosage penicillin and treatment for vascular collapse.

157 (a) Striae atrophicae.
(b) They are a common normal finding at puberty and later.

158 (a) Head lice infestation (pediculosis capitis). Nits (egg cases) are visible in abundance.
(b) Irritation over nape of neck, and secondary bacterial infection will be present.

159 (a) Progeria.
(b) Premature and rapid ageing with onset in infancy.
(c) Patients develop atherosclerosis and die of cardiac or cerebral vascular disease usually in their early teens.

160 (a) Subungual exostosis.
(b) Excision by an orthopaedic surgeon.

161 (a) Contact dermatitis. Due to colophony (rosin) in an adhesive tape.
(b) Patch testing to a battery of chemicals.

162 (a) Langerhans cell histiocytosis (histiocytosis X).
(b) Skin biopsy would be essential. Lymph node and skeletal survey may be indicated.
(c) Prognosis is good with a high rate of spontaneous remission in patients with single system disease (usually bone or lymph node) but management of multisystem disease is controversial with emphasis on immune replacement.

163 (a) Collodion baby.
(b) The shiny transparent but fairly rigid membrane cracks and peels revealing either normal skin or one of the inherited ichthyoses.

164 (a) Cutis marmorata telangiectatica congenita (congenital generalised phlebectasia).
(b) Dilated reticulated venous and capillary channels.
(c) Extends during the first month of life, but tends to improve in childhood.

165, 166 (a) Non-bullous ichthyosiform erythroderma. A rare autosomal recessive disorder. Note the reddened scaly skin.
(b) Emollients are usually the only required therapy. Oral synthetic retinoid therapy does have a place in severe debilitating disease, but side-effects have to be considered.

167 (a) Kerion.
(b) A swollen pustular area containing loose hairs.

168 (a) Pityriasis rubra pilaris. In this child there is a widespread psoriasiform eruption with visible areas of normal skin.
(b) Persistence for months or longer is usual.
(c) Emollients, tar/salicylic acid-containing preparations.

169, 170 (a) Focal dermal hypoplasia (Goltz syndrome). The first illustration shows cheek erythema with depressed scar-like lesions. The second shows visible subcutaneous fat covered only by epidermis.
(b) X-linked dominant, often prenatally lethal in males.

171 (a) Mixed haemangioma.
(b) The superficial capillary portion resolves, but the deeper (cavernous) element may resolve only incompletely.

172 (a) Ingrowing toenail.
(b) Local antiseptics and avoidance of pressure trauma. Surgery can usually be avoided.

173 (a) Lichen nitidus.
(b) Self-limiting, tending to persist for a few months.

174 (a) Acropustulosis of infancy.
(b) Antihistamines are helpful in reducing pruritus. The condition resolves spontaneously in the first 2–3 years of life. Exclude scabies before diagnosing this uncommon condition.

175 (a) Atopic dermatitis. In this child lesions are excoriated and infected.
(b) Mild corticosteroid/antiseptic cream, and a short course of oral antibiotic in view of the infection.

176 (a) Congenital leukaemia. This was acute monoblastic leukaemia. Subcutaneous deposits are visible.
(b) Poor in this form. This infant died of septicaemia despite intensive therapy.

177 (a) Congenital lymphoedema.
(b) Turner's syndrome.

178 (a) Ringworm (tinea pedis).
(b) Soak feet 10 minutes twice daily in potassium permanganate solution (1 in 1000), a topical imidazole cream, and oral griseofulvin.

179 (a) Epidermolytic hyperkeratosis (bullous ichthyosiform erythroderma).
(b) Areas of epidermis peel away shortly after birth leaving readily healing raw areas. The next stage is crops of blisters, which burst and heal rapidly, but have a tendency to secondary infection. Warty hyperkeratosis becomes the dominant feature in time and is strikingly linear in flexures, as in the arm shown.
(c) Careful skin handling, emollients, antiseptics, and antibiotic therapy when necessary. Oral synthetic retinoids may be helpful in selected cases.

180 (a) Salmon patches.
(b) Excellent. Over forehead, glabella, upper eyelids these capillary naevi fade in the first year of life. However, nape of neck lesions ('stork bites') tend to persist, but are usually covered by hair.

181 (a) Hodgkin's disease.
(b) She responded well to chemotherapy.

182 (a) Lichen striatus.
(b) The histology is similar to a chronic dermatitis.

183 (a) Ichthyosis vulgaris.
(b) Small white fine scales usually appear during early childhood. However, shin scales are often large, as in the leg shown. Cubital and popliteal fossae are characteristically spared. Accentuated palmar and plantar skin markings are common.

184 (a) Perioral dermatitis.
(b) There may be multiple causes. This child had an irritant dermatitis associated with dribbling, teething and use of a dummy. Often there is uncertainty in the history regarding the initial lesion, but prescription of topical corticosteroids, particularly potent ones, will certainly perpetuate it.

185 (a) Malignant melanoma. This was the nodular type. Note the more raised upper portion. Rare in children, the condition should not be forgotten in young adults and the incidence is rising.
(b) Adequate excision by an experienced surgeon.

186 (a) Insect bites (due to fleas).
(b) Investigate and deal with source of fleas. Treat with antihistamine and topical corticosteroid/ antibacterial cream.

187 (a) A connective tissue naevus.
(b) Yes, but they may also be a component of an inherited disorder. In this boy a harmless radiological abnormality, osteopoikilosis ('spotted bones') was present, comprising the autosomal dominant Buschke-Ollendorff syndrome.

188 (a) Ecthyma. This is an ulcerative pyoderma.
(b) *Streptococcus pyogenes* and/or *Staphylococcus aureus*.
(c) Oral phenoxymethylpenicillin (Penicillin V) is usually effective.

189 (a) Physiological hair loss.
(b) At term occipital hair roots enter telogen and hairs are therefore shed a few months later. The trauma of both head pressure and movement may contribute to the loss.
(c) Excellent.

190 (a) Hereditary angioedema.
(b) Autosomal dominant.
(c) Affected individuals cannot synthesize normally functioning C1 inhibitor.
(d) With purified C1 inhibitor.

191, 192 (a) Lymphangioma circumscriptum.
(b) At birth or in childhood.
(c) Conservative.

INDEX

numular eczema —
oval shaped lesions
Kinalog